The Chemistry of Food and Nutrition

A. W. Duncan

PREFACE.

The first edition of 1884 contained but 5 pages of type; the second of 1898, 14 pages. Only by conciseness has it been possible to give even a summary of the principles of dietetics within the limit or this pamphlet. Should there appear in places an abruptness or incompleteness of treatment, these limitations must be my excuse.

Those who wish to thoroughly study the science of food are referred to the standard work, "Food and Dietetics," by Dr. R. Hutchison (E. Arnold, 16s.). The effects of purin bodies in producing illness has been patiently and thoroughly worked out by Dr. Alexander Haig. Students are referred to his "Uric Acid, an epitome of the subject" (J. & A. Churchhill, 1904, 2s.6d.), or to his larger work on "Uric Acid." An able scientific summary of investigations on purins, their chemical and pathological properties, and the quantities in foods will be found in "The Purin Bodies of Food Stuffs," by Dr. I. Walker Hall (Sherratt & Hughes, Manchester, 1903, 4s.6d.). The U.S. Department of Agriculture has made a large number of elaborate researches on food and nutrition. My thanks are due to Mr. Albert Broadbent, the Secretary of the Vegetarian Society, for placing some of their bulletins in my hands, and for suggestions and help. He has also written several useful popular booklets on food of a very practical character, at from a penny to threepence each.

Popular literature abounds in unsound statements on food. It is unfortunate that many ardent workers in the cause of health are lacking in scientific knowledge, especially of physiology and chemistry. By their immature and sweeping statements from the platform and press, they often bring discredit on a good cause. Matters of health must be primarily based on experience and we must bear in mind that each person can at the most have full knowledge of himself alone, and to a less degree of his family and intimates. The general rules of health are applicable to all alike, but not in their details. Owing to individual imperfections of constitution, difference of temperament and environment, there is danger when one man attempts to measure others by his own standard.

For the opinions here expressed I only must be held responsible, and not the Society publishing the pamphlet.

Vegetarians, generally, place the humane as the highest reason for their practice, though the determining cause of the change from a flesh diet has been in most cases bad health.

A vegetarian may be defined as one who abstains from all animals as food. The term animal is used in its proper scientific sense (comprising insects, molluscs, crustaceans, fish, etc.). Animal products are not excluded, though they are not considered really necessary. They are looked upon as a great convenience, whilst free from nearly all the objections appertaining to flesh food.

A.W.D.

The Chemistry of Food and Nutrition

By A.W. Duncan, F.C.S.

We may define a food to be any substance which will repair the functional waste of the body, increase its growth, or maintain the heat, muscular, and nervous energy. In its most comprehensive sense, the oxygen of the air is a food; as although it is admitted by the lungs, it passes into the blood, and there re-acts upon the other food which has passed through the stomach. It is usual, however, to restrict the term food to such nutriment as enters the body by the intestinal canal. Water is often spoken of as being distinct from food, but for this there is no sufficient reason.

Many popular writers have divided foods into flesh-formers, heat-givers, and bone-formers. Although attractive from its simplicity, this classification will not bear criticism. Flesh-formers are also heat-givers. Only a portion of the mineral matter goes to form bone.

CLASS I.—INORGANIC COMPOUNDS.
 Sub-class 1. Water. 2. Mineral Matter or Salts.

CLASS II—ORGANIC COMPOUNDS.
 1. Non-Nitrogeneous or Ternary Compounds. *a* Carbohydrates.
  b Oils. *c* Organic Acids.
 2. Nitrogenous Compounds. *a* Proteids. *b* Osseids.

CLASS III.—NON-NUTRITIVES, FOOD ADJUNCTS AND DRUGS.
 Essential Oils, Alkaloids, Extractives, Alcohol, &c.

These last are not strictly foods, if we keep to the definition already given; but they are consumed with the true foods or nutrients, comprised in the other two classes, and cannot well be excluded from consideration.

Water forms an essential part of all the tissues of the body. It is the solvent and carrier of other substances.

Mineral Matter or Salts, is left as an ash when food is thoroughly burnt. The most important salts are calcium phosphate, carbonate and fluoride, sodium chloride, potassium phosphate and chloride, and compounds of magnesium, iron and silicon.

Mineral matter is quite as necessary for plant as for animal life, and is therefore present in all food, except in the case of some highly-prepared ones, such as sugar, starch and oil. Children require a good proportion of calcium phosphate for the growth of their bones, whilst adults require less. The outer part of the grain of cereals is the richest in mineral constituents, white flour and rice are deficient. Wheatmeal and oatmeal are especially recommended for the quantity of phosphates and other salts contained in them. Mineral matter is necessary not only for the bones but for every tissue of the body.

When haricots are cooked, the liquid is often thrown away, and the beans served nearly dry, or with parsley or other sauce. Not only is the food less tasty but important saline constituents are lost. The author has made the following experiments:—German whole lentils, Egyptian split red lentils and medium haricot beans were soaked all night (16 hours) in just sufficient cold water to keep them covered. The water was poured off and evaporated, the residue heated in the steam-oven to perfect dryness and weighed. After pouring off the water, the haricots were boiled in more water until thoroughly cooked, the liquid being kept as low as possible. The liquid was poured off as clear as possible, from the haricots, evaporated and dried. The ash was taken in each case, and the alkalinity of the water-soluble ash was calculated as potash (K_2O). The quantity of water which could be poured off was with the German lentils, half as much more than the original weight of the pulse; not quite as much could be poured off the others.

	G. Lentils.	E. Lentils.	Haricots.	Cooked H.
Proportion of liquid	1.5	1.25	1.20	—
Soluble dry matter	0.97	3.38	1.43	7.66 per cent.
Ash	0.16	0.40	0.28	1.26 " "
Alkalinity as K_2O	0.02	0.082	0.084	0.21 " "

The loss on soaking in cold water, unless the water is preserved, is seen to be considerable. The split lentils, having had the protecting skin removed, lose most. In every case the ash contained a good deal of phosphate and lime. Potatoes are rich in important potash salts; by boiling a large quantity is lost, by steaming less and by baking in the skins, scarcely any. The flavour is also much better after baking.

The usual addition of common salt (sodium-chloride) to boiled potatoes is no proper substitute for the loss of their natural saline constituents. Natural and properly cooked foods are so rich in sodium chloride and other salts that the addition of common salt is unnecessary. An excess of the latter excites thirst and spoils the natural flavour of the food. It is the custom, especially in restaurants, to add a large quantity of salt to pulse, savoury food, potatoes and soups. Bakers' brown bread is usually very salt, and sometimes white is also. In some persons much salt causes irritation of the skin, and the writer has knowledge of the salt food of vegetarian restaurants causing or increasing dandruff. As a rule, fondness for salt is an acquired taste, and after its discontinuance for a time, food thus flavoured becomes unpalatable.

Organic Compounds are formed by living organisms (a few can also be produced by chemical means). They are entirely decomposed by combustion.

The **Non-Nitrogenous Organic Compounds** are commonly called carbon compounds or heat-producers, but these terms are also descriptive of the nitrogenous compounds. These contain carbon, hydrogen and oxygen only, and furnish by their oxidation or combustion in the body the necessary heat, muscular and nervous energy. The final product of their combustion is water and carbon dioxide (carbonic acid gas).

The **Carbohydrates** comprise starch, sugar, gum, mucilage, pectose, glycogen, &c.; cellulose and woody fibre are carbohydrates, but are little capable of digestion. They contain hydrogen and oxygen in the proportion to form water, the carbon alone being available to produce heat by combustion. Starch is the most widely distributed food. It is insoluble in water, but when cooked is readily digested and absorbed by the body. Starch is readily converted into sugar, whether in plants or animals, during digestion. There are many kinds of sugar, such as grape, cane and milk sugars.

The **Oils and Fats** consist of the same elements as the carbohydrates, but the hydrogen is in larger quantity than is necessary to form water, and this surplus is available for the production of energy. During their combustion in the body they produce nearly two-and-a-quarter times (4 : 8.9 = 2.225) as much heat as the carbohydrates; but if eaten in more than small quantities, they are not easily digested, a portion passing away by the intestines. The fat in the body is not solely dependent upon the quantity consumed as food, as an animal may become quite fat on food containing none. A moderate quantity favours digestion and the bodily health. In cold weather more should be taken. In the Arctic regions the Esquimaux consume enormous quantities. Nuts are generally rich in oil. Oatmeal contains more than any of the other cereals (27 analyses gave from 8 to 12.3 per cent.)

The most esteemed and dearest oil is Almond. What is called Peach-kernel oil (Oleum Amygdalæ Persicæ), but which in commerce includes the oil obtained from plum and apricot stones, is almost as tasteless and useful, whilst it is considerably cheaper. It is a very agreeable and useful food. It is often added to, as an adulterant, or substituted for the true Almond oil. The best qualities of Olive oil are much esteemed, though they are not as agreeable to English taste as the oil previously mentioned. The best qualities are termed Virgin, Extra Sublime and Sublime. Any that has been exposed for more than a short time to the light and heat of a shop window should be rejected, as the flavour is affected. It should be kept in a cool place. Not only does it vary much in freedom from acid and rancidity, but is frequently adulterated. Two other cheaper oils deserve mention. The "cold-drawn" Arachis oil (pea-nut or earth-nut oil) has a pleasant flavour, resembling that of kidney beans. The "cold-drawn" Sesamé oil has an agreeable taste, and is considered equal to Olive oil for edible purposes. The best qualities are rather difficult to obtain; those usually sold being much inferior to Peach-kernel and Olive oils. Cotton-seed oil is the cheapest of the edible ones. Salad oil, not sold under any descriptive name, is usually refined Cotton-seed oil, with perhaps a little Olive oil to impart a richer flavour.

The solid fats sold as butter and lard substitutes, consist of deodorised cocoanut oil, and they are excellent for cooking purposes. It is claimed that biscuits, &c., made from them may be kept for a much longer period, without showing any trace of rancidity, than if butter or lard had been used. They are also to be had agreeably flavoured by admixture with almond, walnut, &c., "cream."

The better quality oils are quite as wholesome as the best fresh butter, and better than most butter as sold. Bread can be dipped into the oil, or a little solid vegetable fat spread on it. The author prefers to pour a little Peach-kernel oil upon some ground walnut kernels (or other ground nuts in themselves rich in oil), mix with a knife to a suitable consistency and spread upon the bread. Pine-kernels are very oily, and can be used in pastry in the place of butter or lard.

Whenever oils are mentioned, without a prefix, the fixed or fatty oils are always understood. The volatile or essential oils are a distinct class. Occasionally, the fixed oils are called hydrocarbons, but hydrocarbon oils are quite different and consist of carbon and hydrogen alone. Of these, petroleum is incapable of digestion, whilst others are poisonous.

Vegetable Acids are composed of the same three elements and undergo combustion into the same compounds as the carbohydrates. They rouse the appetite, stimulate digestion, and finally form carbonates in combination with the alkalies, thus increasing the alkalinity of the blood. The chief vegetable acids are: malic acid, in the apple, pear, cherry, &c.; citric acid, in the lemon, lime, orange, gooseberry, cranberry, strawberry, raspberry, &c.; tartaric acid, in the grape, pineapple, &c.

Some place these under Class III. or food adjuncts. Oxalic acid (except when in the insoluble state of calcium oxalate), and several other acids are poisonous.

Proteids or Albuminoids are frequently termed flesh-formers. They are composed of nitrogen, carbon, hydrogen, oxygen, and a small quantity of sulphur, and are extremely complex bodies. Their chief function is to form flesh in the body; but without previously forming it, they may be transformed into fat or merely give rise to heat. They form the essential part of every living cell.

Proteids are excreted from the body as water, carbon dioxide, urea, uric acid, sulphates, &c.

The principal proteids of animal origin have their corresponding proteids in the vegetable kingdom. Some kinds, whether of animal or vegetable origin, are more easily digested than others. They have the same physiological value from whichever kingdom they are derived.

The **Osseids** comprise ossein, gelatin, cartilage, &c., from bone, skin, and connective issue. They approach the proteids in composition, but unlike them they cannot form flesh or fulfil the same purpose in nutrition. Some food chemists wish to call the osseids, albuminoids; what were formerly termed albuminoids to be always spoken of as proteids only.

Jellies are of little use as food; not only is this because of the low nutritive value of gelatin, but also on account of the small quantity which is mixed with a large proportion of water.

The **Vegetable Kingdom** is the prime source of all organic food; water, and to a slight extent salts, form the only food that animals can derive directly from the inorganic kingdom. When man consumes animal food—a sheep for example—he is only consuming a portion of the food which that sheep obtained from grass, clover, turnips, &c. All the proteids of the flesh once existed as proteids in the vegetables; some in exactly the same chemical form.

Flesh contains no starch or sugar, but a small quantity of glycogen. The fat in an animal is derived from the carbohydrates, the fats and the proteids of the vegetables consumed. The soil that produced the herbage, grain and roots consumed by cattle, in most cases could have produced food capable of direct utilisation by man. By passing the product of the soil through animals there is an enormous economic loss, as the greater part of that food is dissipated in maintaining the life and growth; little remains as flesh when the animal is delivered into the hands of the butcher. Some imagine that flesh food is more easily converted into flesh and blood in our bodies and is consequently more valuable than similar constituents in vegetables, but such is not the case. Fat, whether from flesh or from vegetables is digested in the same manner. The proteids of flesh, like those of vegetables, are converted into peptone by the digestive juices—taking the form of a perfectly diffusible liquid—otherwise they could not be absorbed and utilised by the body. Thus the products of digestion of both animal and vegetable proteids and fats are the same. Formerly, proteid matter was looked upon as the most valuable part of the food, and a large proportion was thought necessary for hard work. It was thought to be required, not only for the construction of the muscle substance, but to be utilised in proportion to muscular exertion. These views are now known to be wrong. A comparatively small quantity of proteid matter, such as is easily obtained from vegetable food, is ample for the general needs of the body. Increased muscular exertion requires but a slight increase of this food constituent. It is the carbohydrates, or carbohydrates and fats that should be eaten in larger quantity, as these are the main source of muscular energy. The fact that animals, capable of the most prolonged and powerful exertion, thrive on vegetables of comparatively low proteid value, and that millions of the strongest races have subsisted on what most Englishmen would consider a meagre vegetarian diet, should have been sufficient evidence against the earlier view.

A comparison of flesh and vegetable food, shows in flesh an excessive quantity of proteid matter, a very small quantity of glycogen (the animal equivalent of starch and sugar) and a variable quantity of fat. Vegetable food differs much, but as a rule it contains a much smaller quantity of proteid matter, a large proportion of starch and sugar and a small quantity of fat. Some vegetable foods, particularly nuts, contain much fat.

Investigation of the digestive processes has shown that the carbohydrates and fats entail little strain on the system; their ultimate products are water and carbon dioxide, which are easily disposed of. The changes which the proteids undergo in the body are very complicated. There is ample provision in the body for their digestion, metabolism, and final rejection, when taken in moderate quantity, as is the case in a dietary of vegetables. The proteids in the human body, after fulfilling their purpose, are in part expelled in the same way as the carbohydrates; but the principal part, including all the nitrogen, is expelled by the kidneys in the form of urea (a very soluble substance), and a small quantity of uric acid in the form of quadurates.

There is reciprocity between the teeth and digestive organs of animals and their natural food. The grasses, leaves, &c., which are consumed by the herbivora, contain a large proportion of cellulose and woody tissue. Consequently, the food is bulky; it is but slowly disintegrated and the nutritious matter liberated and digested. The cellulose appears but slightly acted upon by the digestive juices. The herbivora possess capacious stomachs and the intestines are very long. The carnivora have simpler digestive organs and short intestines. Even they consume substances which leave much indigestible residue, such as skin, ligaments and bones, but civilised man, when living on a flesh dietary removes as much of such things as possible. The monkeys, apes, and man (comprised in the order *Primates* have a digestive canal intermediate in complexity and in length to the herbivora and carnivora. A certain quantity of indigestible matter is necessary for exciting peristaltic action of the bowels. The carnivora with their short intestinal canal need the least, the frugivora more, and the herbivora a much larger quantity. The consumption by man of what is commonly called concentrated food is the cause of the constipation to which flesh-eating nations are subject. Most of the pills and other nostrums which are used in enormous quantities contain aloes or other drugs which stimulate the action of the intestines.

Highly manufactured foods, from which as much as possible of the non-nutritious matter has been removed is often advocated, generally by those interested in its sale. Such food would be advantageous only if it were possible to remove or modify a great part of our digestive canal (we are omitting from consideration certain diseased conditions, when such foods may be useful). The eminent physiologist and bacteriologist, Elie Metchnikoff, has given it as his opinion that much of man's digestive organs is not only useless but often productive of derangement and disease. In several cases where it has been necessary, in consequence of serious disease, to remove the entire stomach or a large part of the intestines, the digestive functions have been perfectly performed. It is not that our organs are at fault, but our habits of life differ from that of our progenitors. In past times, when a simple dietary in which flesh food formed little or no part, and to-day, in those countries where one wholly or nearly all derived from vegetable sources and simply prepared is the rule, diseases of the digestive organs are rare. The Englishman going to a tropical country and partaking largely of flesh and alcohol, suffers from disease of the liver and other organs, to which the natives and the few of his own countrymen, living in accordance with natural laws are strangers.

Indigestible Matter—Food is never entirely digested. As a reason against confining ourselves solely to vegetable food, it has been stated that such is less perfectly digested than animal food and that it therefore throws more work on the digestive organs. It is also urged that on this account a greater quantity of vegetable food is required. We have shown elsewhere that, on the contrary, vegetarians are satisfied with a smaller amount of food. Man requires a small quantity of woody fibre or cellulose in his food to stimulate intestinal action and prevent constipation.

It is difficult to determine how much of a food is unassimilated in the body. This is for the reason of the intestinal refuse consisting not only of undigested food, but also of residues of the digestive juices, mucus and epithelial debris. These latter have been shown to amount to from one-third to one-half of the whole of the fæces, which is much more than had previously been supposed.

John Goodfellow has shown that of very coarse wholemeal bread quite 14 per cent. was undigested, whilst bread made from ordinary grade wholemeal showed 12.5 per cent. Such a method of analysis was adopted as it was believed would exclude other than the food waste. The experiments were made on a person who was eating nothing but the bread. It seems probable that a smaller proportion would have remained unassimilated had the bread not formed the sole food. It is advisable that wheatmeal he ground as finely as possible, the coarse is not only to a less extent assimilated but apt to irritate the bowels. Notwithstanding that fine white bread gave only 4.2 per cent. and a coarse white bread 4.9 per cent. of waste, a fine wheatmeal bread is more economical as the same quantity of wheat produces a greater weight of flour richer in proteid and mineral matter. From a large number of experiments with man, it has been calculated that of proteids there is digested when animal food is eaten 98 per cent., from cereals and sugars 8 per cent., from vegetables and fruits 80 per cent. The difference between the proportions digested of the other food constituents was much less. Although there is here a theoretical advantage in favour of animal food, there are other considerations of far more importance than a little undigestible waste. The main question is one of health. In some dietary experiments of a girl aged 7, living upon a fruit diet, of whom we have given some particulars elsewhere, Professor Jaffa gives the following particulars. During the ten days trial the percentages absorbed were proteids 82.5, fat 86.9, nitrogen free extract 96, crude fibre 80, ash 5.7, heat of combustion in calories 86.7. He says, "generally speaking, the food was quite thoroughly assimilated, the coefficients of digestibility being about the same as are found in an ordinary mixed diet. It is interesting to note that 80 per cent. of the crude fibre appeared to be digested. The results of a number of foreign experiments on the digestibility of crude fibre by man are from 30 to 91.4 per cent., the former value being from mixed wheat and rye, and the latter in a diet made of rice, vegetables and meat."

TABLE OF ANALYSIS OF FOOD.

	Proteids.	Fat.	Carbohydrates.	Ash.	Cellulose.	Refuse.	Water.	Calories.	N't'nt Ratio
Wholemeal, G.	14.9	1.6	66.2	1.7	1.6	...	14.0	1577	4.68
Fine Flour, G.	9.3	0.8	76.5	0.7	0.7	...	12.0	1629	8·4
Medium Flour, G....	12.1	0.9	72.2	0.9	0.9	...	13.0	1606	6.13
Bread, Wh'lem'l, G.	12.2	1.2	43.5	1.3	1.8	...	40.0	1086	3.8
,, White, G....	7.5	0.8	53.8	0.9	...	...	37.0	1174	7.4
Macaroni, U.........	13.4	0.9	74·1	1.3	...	...	10.3	1665	5.67
Oatmeal, D.	14.8	9.6	63.3	2.2	1.4	...	8.7	1858	5.72
Maize, American, S.	10.0	4.25	71.75	1.5	1.75	...	10.75	1700	8.12
Rice, husked, U. ...	8.0	0.3	79.0	0.4	...	...	12.3	1630	10.0
Rye Flour, U.	6.8	0.9	78.3	0.7	0.4	...	12.9	1620	11.8
Barley, Pearl, C. ...	6.2	1.3	76.0	1.1	0.8	...	14.6	1584	12.7
Buckwheat Flour,U.	6.4	1.2	77.9	0.9	...	...	13.6	1619	12.6
Soy Bean, C.	35.3	18.9	26.0	4.6	4.2	...	11.0	1938	1.93
Pea-nut, C............	24.5	50.0	11.7	1.8	4.5	...	7.5	2783	5.2
Lentils, U............	25.7	1.0	59.2	5.7	...	...	8.4	1621	2.4
Peas, dried, U.	24.6	1.0	62.0	2.9	4.5	...	9.5	1655	2.6
Peas, green, E.U....	7.0	0.5	15.2	1.0	1.7	...	74.6	465	2.3
Haricots, C.	23.0	2.3	52.3	2.9	5.5	...	14.0	1463	2.5
Walnuts, fresh k., C.	12.5	31.6	8.9	1.7	0.8	...	44.5	1565	6.33
Walnut kernels	21.4	54.1	15.2	2.9	1.4	...	5.0	2964	6.33
Filberts,fresh ker.,C.	8.4	28.5	11.1	1.5	2.5	...	48.0	1506	8.9
Tomatoes, U.........	1.2	0.2	3.5	0.6	0.5	...	94.0	105	3.3
Grapes, U.	1.0	1.2	10.1	0.4	4.3	25	58.0	335	12.8
Apples, E.U.	0.4	0.5	13.0	0.3	1.2	(25)	84.6	290	35.3
Raisins, E.U.........	2.6	3.3	76.1	3.4	...	(10)	14.6	1605	32.0
Dates, E.U.	2.1	2.8	78.4	1.3	...	(10)	15.4	1615	40.0
Banana, C.D........	1.71	...	20.13	0.71	1.74	...	75.7	406	11.7
Banana Flour, P. ...	3.13	1.73	82.4	5.93	1.21	...	5.6	1664	27.5
Potatoes, K.	1.9	0.2	20.7	1.0	0.7	..	75.7	429	11.0
Turnips, E............	1.3	0.2	6.8	0.8	1.3	(30)	89.6	159	5.57
Onions, E.U.........	1.6	0.3	9.1	0.6	0.8	(10)	87.6	225	6.1
Cabbage, E.U.	1.6	0.3	4.5	1.0	1.1	(15)	91.5	123	3.23
Asparagus, U.	1.5	0.1	2.3	1.2	0.5	...	94.4	85	1.7
Celery, E.U.	1.1	0.1	3.3	1.0	...	(20)	94.5	85	3.2
Mushrooms, U.	3.5	0.4	6.8	1.2	...	...	88.1	210	2.2
Tapioca, U...	0.4	0.1	88.0	0.1	...	...	11.4	1650	220
Sugar	...	...	100	...	...	...	...	1860	...
Oil	...	100	...	...	...	...	...	4220	...
Milk	3.6	3.7	4.6	0.73	...	...	87.4	309	3.56
Butter, fresh	0.8	83.5	1.5	0.2	...	...	14.0	3566	234
Cheese, U.	25.9	33.7	2.4	3.8	...	...	34.2	1950	3.0
Hen's Eggs, U......	11.9	9.3	...	0.9	...	11.2	65.5	635	1.74
Beef, loin, U.........	16.4	16.9	...	0.9	...	13.3	52.9	1020	2.3
Beef,loin,edible p.,U	19.0	19.1	...	1.0	...	...	61.3	1155	2.3
Mutton, shoulder, U.	13.7	17.1	...	0.7	...	22.1	46.8	975	2.77
Pork, Ham, U.	14.3	29.7	...	0.8	...	10.3	45.1	1520	4.6
Bacon, smoked, U.	9.5	59.4	...	4.5	...	8.7	18.4	2685	13.9
Fowl, U.	13.7	12.3	...	0.7	...	25.9	47.1	775	2.0
Goose, U.	13.4	29.8	...	0.7	...	17.6	38.5	1505	4.9
Cod, dressed, U......	11.1	0.2	...	0.8	...	29.9	58.5	215	0.04
Mackerel, whole, U.	10.2	4.2	...	0.7	...	44.7	40.4	365	9.15
Oysters, L............	8.75	0.92	8.09	2.4	...	...	79.8	352	1.16

NOTES ON THE TABLE OF ANALYSIS.—Under calories are shown kilo-calories per pound of food. In the analysis marked U the crude fibre or cellulose is included with the carbo-hydrate, the figures being those given in Atwater's table. He has found that from 30 to 91 per cent. of the crude fibre was digested, according to the kind of food. The term fibre or cellulose in analytical tables is not a very definite one. It depends upon the details of the method of analysis. In the analyses other than U, the cellulose is excluded in calculating the calories. Nutrient ratio is the proportion of the sum of the carbo-hydrate and fat, compared with the proteid as 1. The fat has first been multiplied by 2.225 to bring it to the same nutrient value as the carbo-hydrate.

U indicates that the analyses are taken from the United States Department of Agriculture Experimental Station, Bulletin 28, the tests being chiefly made by Dr. W.O. Atwater, or under his direction. They are average analyses of several samples. The refuse consists of such parts as are rejected in preparing the food; the outer leaves, skin, stalk, seeds, &c., of vegetables; the shell of eggs; the bone, &c., of meat. E, indicates that the edible portion only of the food has been analysed, and under refuse, in brackets, is shown the quantity rejected before the analysis was made.

There is considerable variation in the same kind of food, according to the variety of seed and conditions of growth &c., especially is this the case with wheat and flour; whenever it has been possible the average of the analyses of many samples have been given. The method of analysis has not always been uniform, frequently the cellulose is included with the carbo-hydrates, and the proteid sometimes includes a very appreciable quantity of non-proteid nitrogenous matter. This is the case in the analysis of the mushrooms. G.—Analyses are by John Goodfellow; it will be noticed that the wheatmeal bread is not made from the same flour as the whole-meal. D.—B. Dyer, average of 19 fine and coarse oatmeals. S, from U.S. Cons. Reports, 1899. C.—A.H. Church. The walnut kernels are in the dried condition as purchased; originally of the same composition as shewn in the fresh kernels. C.D.—Cavendish or Figi variety of banana, analysis by D.W.M. Doherty, N.S. Wales. P.—A. Petermann, U.S. Cons. Banana flour, *musca paradisiaca* variety. This is widely used in Central America. The flour is from the unripe fruit, and contains starch 45.7 per cent.; on ripening the starch is converted into sugar. K.—Konig, mean of 90 analysis. Milk:—Average of many thousand analyses of the pure. Butter.—Made without salt. L, from the "Lancet," 1903, I, p. 72. Oysters at 2/6 per dozen. The 8.09 per cent. includes 0.91 glycogen (animal starch). The shell was of course excluded, also the liquid in the shell. Apples. —The refuse includes seeds, skin, &c., and such edible portion as is wasted in cutting them away; the analysis was made on the rest.

Cookery.—Flesh is easier to digest raw. A few, on the advice of their doctors, eat minced raw flesh, raw beef juice and even fresh warm blood. Such practice is abhorrent to every person of refinement. Cooking lessens the offensive appearance and qualities of flesh and changes the flavour; thorough cooking also destroys any parasites that may be present. Raw flesh is more stimulating to the animal passions, and excites ferocity in both man and animals. If the old argument was valid, that as flesh is much nearer in composition and quality to our own flesh and tissues, it is therefore our best food, we do wrong in coagulating the albuminoids, hardening the muscle substance and scorching it by cooking.

Fruits when ripe and in good condition are best eaten raw; cooking spoils the flavour. Food requiring mastication and encouraging insalivation is the best. Food is frequently made too sloppy or liquid, and is eaten too hot, thus favouring indigestion and decay of the teeth. The cereals and pulses can only with difficulty be eaten raw. When cooked in water the starch granules swell and break up, the plant cells are ruptured, the fibres are separated and the nutritious matter rendered easy of digestion. The flavour is greatly improved. Cooking increases our range and variety of food. The civilised races use it to excess and over-season their dishes, favouring over-eating.

If baking powders are used they should only be of the best makes. They should be composed of sodium bicarbonate and tartaric acid, in such correct proportions that upon the addition of water only sodium tartrate and carbon dioxide (carbonic acid) should result. Some powders contain an excess of sodium bicarbonate. Self-raising flours should be avoided. They are commonly composed of—in addition to sodium bicarbonate—acid calcium phosphate, calcium superphosphate and calcium sulphate. Common baking powders often consist of the same ingredients, and sometimes also of magnesia and alum. These are often made and sold by ignorant men, whose sole object is to make money. Calcium superphosphate and acid calcium phosphate very frequently contain arsenic, and as the cheap commercial qualities are often used there is danger in this direction. A good formula for baking powder is, tartaric acid 8 ozs., sodium bicarbonate 9 ozs., rice flour 10 to 20 ozs. The last is added to baking powders to improve the keeping quality and to add bulk. The ingredients must be first carefully dried, the sodium bicarbonate at not too high a temperature or it decomposes, and then thoroughly mixed; this must be preserved in well closed and dry bottles. Another formula, which is slow rising and well adapted for pastry, is sodium bicarbonate 4 ozs., cream of tartar 9 ozs., rice flour about 14 ozs. Custard powders consist of starch, colouring and flavouring. Egg powders are similar to baking powders but contain yellow colouring. Little objection can be taken to them if they are coloured with saffron; turmeric would do if it were not that it gives a slightly unpleasant taste. Artificial colouring matters or coal tar derivatives are much used, several of these are distinctly poisonous.

Drinks.—It is better not to drink during eating, or insalivation may be interfered with; a drink is better taken at the end of a meal. The practice of washing down food with hot tea is bad. The refreshing nature of a cup of hot tea, coffee, or cocoa is to a very great extent due to the warmth of the water. The benefit is felt at once, before the alkaloid can enter the blood stream and stimulate the nerve centres. Hot water, not too hot to cause congestion of the mucous membrane, is one of the best drinks. When the purity of the water supply is doubtful, there is advantage in first bringing it to the boil, as pathogenic bacteria are destroyed. Some find it beneficial to drink a cup of hot water the first thing in the morning; this cleanses the stomach from any accumulation of mucus.

If fruit, succulent vegetables, or cooked food, containing much water be freely used, and there be little perspiration, it is possible to do without drinking; but there is danger of taking insufficient water to hold freely in solution the waste products excreted by the body.

Aerated drinks, except a very few of the best, and non-alcoholic beers and wines, are generally unwholesome, from their containing preservatives, foaming powders, artificial flavourings, &c.

Stimulants.—Tea and coffee contain an alkaloid theine, besides volatile oils, tannin, &c. Cocoa contains the milder alkaloid, theobromine. They stimulate the heart and nervous systems; tea and coffee have also a diuretic effect. Formerly they were erroneously thought to lessen tissue waste. These alkaloids, being purins, are open to the general objections named elsewhere. Stimulants do not impart energy or force of any kind, but only call forth reserve strength by exciting the heart, nervous system, &c., to increased activity. This is followed by a depression which is as great, generally greater, than the previous stimulation. Except, perhaps, as an occasional medicine, stimulants, should be avoided. Analysis of cocoa shows a good proportion of proteids and a very large quantity of fat. The claim that it is a valuable and nutritious food would only be true if it could be eaten in such quantities as are other foods (bread, fruits, &c.). Were this attempted, poisoning would result from the large quantity of alkaloid. The food value of half a spoonful or thereabouts of cocoa is insignificant. Certain much advertised cocoa mixtures are ridiculous in their pretentions, unscientific in preparation, and often injurious.

Cereals.—The most valuable is wheat, from its proteid being chiefly in the form known as gluten. From its tenacity, gluten enables a much better loaf to be produced from wheat than from any other cereal. The outer part of the grain is the richest in mineral matter and proteid. Wheatmeal bread shows a considerably higher proteid value than white. A large proportion of the proteid in the outer coats of the wheat berry is, however, not digested, and in some experiments the waste has been enough to quite nullify its seeming advantage over white bread. Coarsely ground, sharp branny particles in bread irritate the intestines, and cause excessive waste of nutriment; but finely ground wheatmeal is free from this objection, and is beneficial in preventing constipation. The comparative value of white and brown bread has been much discussed; it depends both on the quality of the bread and the condition of the digestive organs. Experiments on the digestion of bread and other things, have often been made on persons unaccustomed to such foods, or the foods have been given in excessive quantity. To those accustomed to it good wheatmeal bread is much pleasanter, more satisfying, and better flavoured than white; indeed, the latter is described as insipid. Most bakers' bread is of unsatisfactory quality. Flour and bread contain very little fat, the absence of which is considered a defect. This is remedied by the addition of butter, fat or oil, or by nuts, &c., which are rich in oil. These may be mixed with the flour prior to cooking, or used afterwards.

Oats contain a substance called avenin, apparently an alkaloid, which has an irritating action; the quantity is variable. It is to this that the so-called heating effect of oatmeal on some persons is due.

Prepared Cereals or Breakfast Foods.—Analyses were made of 34 of these cereal preparations by Weems and Ellis (Iowa State College Agricultural

Bulletin, 1904). They report that the foods possess no nutritive value in excess of ordinary food materials; that the claim made for many pre-digested foods are valueless, and no reliance can be placed on the statement that they are remedies for any disease.

Oatmeal and other cereals are sold in packets as being partially cooked. We do not doubt that they have been subjected to a dry heat, but this has scarcely any effect on their starch and other constituents. The difference is a mechanical one. In rolled oats the grains are so cracked and broken, that on boiling with water, the water readily penetrates and more quickly cooks them throughout. There are other prepared cereal foods, but we doubt whether they are thoroughly cooked after the short boiling directed on the labels. They are a great convenience where it is difficult to get the time necessary for cooking the ordinary cereals. Coarsely ground wheat is too irritating when made into porridge, but there are some granulated wheats sold in packets, which are quite suitable. The Ralston breakfast food is excellent. They are rich in the phosphates and salts, found in the outer part of the grain. One cereal preparation called Grape Nuts, has had its starch converted into maltose and dextrin (maltose being a sugar), by a scientific application of the diastase of the grain. It is consequently easier of digestion and requires no cooking. It is beneficial for some forms of indigestion. There are several competing foods of less merit, the starch being less perfectly changed; one at least of which is objectionably salt. Properly cooked starch is readily digested by healthy persons, and for them malted food is of no special value.

Pulse, or Legumes, includes haricots and other beans, peas and lentils. The proteid contained is that variety known as legumin, which is either the same, or is closely allied, to the casein of milk and cheese. Pulse is very rich in proteid, the dried kinds in general use, contain 24 or 25 per cent. The richest is the soy-bean, which is used in China and Japan, it contains 35 per cent., besides 19 per cent. of fat. Pulse requires thorough cooking, haricots taking the longest time. Split lentils are cooked sooner, and are better digested; this is chiefly due to the removal of the skins. The haricots, bought from small grocers who have a slow sale, are often old, and will not cook tender. Pulse is best adapted to the labouring classes; the sedentary should eat it sparingly, it is liable to cause flatulence or accumulation of gas in the intestines, and constipation. Haricots are easier to digest when mashed and mixed with other food. Pulse was formerly stated to leave much undigested residue. Recent experiments have shown that it is satisfactorily digested under favourable conditions. Strümpell found beans in their skins to leave a large proportion of proteid matter unabsorbed. Lentil meal mixed with other food was digested in a perfectly satisfactory manner. Another experimenter (Rubner) found that when even the very large quantity of 1-1/8 pound of dried split peas per day were eaten, only 17 per cent. of proteid matter was unabsorbed, which compares very well with the 11 per cent. of proteid left from a macaroni diet, with which the same man was fed at another time. Had a reasonable quantity of peas been eaten per day, the quantity undigested would probably have differed little from that of other foods.

Nuts are, as a rule, very rich in oil and contain a fair proportion of proteid; when well masticated they are a very valuable food. Walnuts are one of the best, and the kernels can be purchased shelled, thus avoiding much trouble. They can be finely ground in a nut-mill and used for several purposes, mixed in the proportion of about two ounces to the pound of wheatmeal they produce a rich flavoured bread. They can also he used in sweet cakes and in rich puddings to increase their food value, lightness and taste. Pine kernels being very oily, can be used with flour in the place of lard or butter.

Fruits are generally looked upon as luxuries, rather than as food capable of supplying a meal or a substantial part of one. They are usually eaten only when the appetite has been appeased by what is considered more substantial fare. Fresh fruits contain a larger proportion of water than nearly all other raw foods, and consequently the proportion of nourishment is small; but we must not despise them on this account. Milk contains as much or more water. Certain foods which in the raw state contain very little water, such as the pulses and cereals when cooked absorb a very large quantity; this is particularly the case in making porridge. Cabbage, cauliflower, Spanish onions and turnips, after cooking contain even 97 per cent. of water. Roast beef contains on an average 48 per cent., and cooked round steak with fat removed 63 per cent. of water. It is customary at meal times to drink water, tea, coffee, beer, wine, &c. When a meal contains any considerable quantity of fresh fruits there need be no desire to drink. Notwithstanding that fruits contain so much water, a dietary consisting of fruits with nuts, to which may be added bread and vegetables, will contain less water than the total quantity usually consumed by a person taking the more customary highly cooked and seasoned foods. An advantage is that the water in fruits is in a wholesome condition, free from the pollution often met with in the water used for drinking purposes. Raw fruits favour mastication, with its consequent advantages, whilst cooked and soft food discourages it. Plums and what are termed stone fruits, if eaten in more than very small quantities, are apt to disagree. Persons with good digestions can take fruit with bread, biscuits and with uncooked foods without any inconvenience. Fruit is more likely to disagree when taken in conjunction with elaborately cooked foods. Many cannot take fruit, especially if it be acid, at the same time as cereal or starchy substances, and the difficulty is said to be greater at the morning's meal. If the indigestion produced is due to the acid of the fruit preventing the saliva acting on the starch, scientific principles would direct that the fruit be eaten quite towards the end of the meal. The same consideration condemns the use of mint sauce, cucumber and vinegar, or pickles, with potatoes and bread, or even mint sauce with green peas. Bananas are an exception, as not interfering with the digestion of starch. Bananas are generally eaten in an unripe condition, white and somewhat mealy; they should be kept until the starch has been converted into sugar, when they are both more pleasant and wholesome. Nuts and fruit go well together. For a portable meal, stoned raisins or other dried fruit and walnut kernels or other nuts are excellent.

What has been called a defect in most fruits, is the fact that the proteid is small in proportion to the other constituents. This has been too much dwelt upon, owing to the prevailing exaggerated idea of the quantity of proteid required. The tomato contains a large proportion, though the water is very high. Bananas, grapes and strawberries contain to each part of proteid from 10 to 12 parts of other solid nutritive constituents (any oil being calculated into starch equivalents); this is termed the nutritive ratio. Although this may seem a small proportion of proteid, there are reasons for believing that it is sufficient. Taking the average of 29 analyses of American apples, a nutritive ratio of 33 was obtained. If it were suggested that life should be sustained on apples alone, this small quantity of proteid would be an insurmountable difficulty. As the addition of nuts or other nutritious food sufficiently increases the proteid, no objection can with justice be made against the use of fruit. A study of our teeth, digestive organs and general structure, and of comparative anatomy, points to fruits, nuts and succulent vegetables as our original diet.

The potash and other salts of the organic acids in fruits tend to keep the blood properly alkaline. Where there is a tendency to the deposition of uric acid in the body, they hinder its formation. Citric, tartaric, malic and other organic acids exist in fruits in combination with potash and other bases, as well as in the free state. The free acids in fruits, when eaten, combine with the alkalies in the intestinal tract, and are absorbed by the body and pass into the blood, not as acids, but as neutral salts. Here they are converted into potassium carbonate or some other carbonate. Fruit acids never make the blood acid but the reverse. Fruit salts and acids are antiscorbutic. Fruits have often proved of the greatest benefit in illness. What is known as the grape cure has been productive of much good. Lemons and oranges have also been of great benefit. Strawberries have been craved for and have proved of the greatest advantage in some extreme cases of illness when more concentrated food could not be endured. Fruit is coming into greater use, especially owing to its better distribution and lessened cost. Fruit is not as cheap as it should be, as it can be produced in great abundance at little cost, and with comparatively little labour. The price paid by the public greatly exceeds the real cost of production. A very large proportion, often the greater part of the cost to the consumer, goes in railway and other rates and in middle-men's profits. It is commonly cheaper to bring fruit from over the sea, including land carriage on either side, than it is to transport English produce from one part of our country to another. English homegrown fruit would be cheaper were it not for the difficulty of buying suitable land at a reasonable price, and the cost of transit. For the production of prime fruit there is a lack of sufficient intelligence, of scientific culture and co-operation.

Vegetables—using the name in its popular sense—contain valuable saline constituents or salts. By the usual method of cooking a large proportion of the salts is lost. It is better to steam than to boil them. The fibrous portion of vegetables is not all digested, but it is useful in stimulating the peristaltic action of the bowels and lessening any tendency to constipation. Vegetables are more especially useful to non-vegetarians to correct the defects of their other food.

The potato belongs to a poisonous order—the *Solanacœ*. There is a little alkaloid in the skin, but this is lost in the cooking. The eyes and sprouting portions contain the most and should be cut out.

Fungi.—There are about a hundred edible species in this country, but many of the fungi are poisonous, some intensely so. It can scarcely be expected that these lowly organised plants, differing so much in their manner of growth from the green or chlorophyll bearing plants, can be particularly nourishing. It is only the fructifying part, which appears above the ground, that is generally eaten. It is of very rapid growth. Of 9 edible fungi of 4 species, obtained in the

Belgrade market, the average amount of water was 89.3 per cent., leaving only 10.7 per cent. of solid matter; the average of fat was 0.55 per cent. The food value of fungi has been greatly over-rated. In most of the analyses given in text-books and elsewhere, the total nitrogen has been multiplied by 6.25 and the result expressed as proteid. The amount of nitrogen in a form useless for the purpose of nutrition is about a third of the whole. Of the remainder or proteid nitrogen, it is said much is not assimilated, sometimes quite half, owing to the somewhat indigestible character of the fungi. An analysis of the common mushroom gave proteids 2.2 per cent., amides (useless nitrogenous compounds) 1.3 per cent., and water 93.7 per cent. The fungi are of inferior nutritive value to many fresh vegetables and are much more expensive. Their chief value is as a flavouring.

Milk and Eggs are permissible in a vegetarian dietary, and as a rule, vegetarians use them. Eggs, with the exception of such as are unfertile, are of course alive; but they have no conscious existence, and cannot be said to suffer any pain on being killed and eaten. An objection to their use as food is, that on an egg and poultry farm, the superfluous male birds are killed, and as the hens become unprofitable layers they are also killed. A similar humane objection applies to the use of cow's milk by man. The calves are deprived of part of their natural food, the deficiency being perhaps made up by unnatural farinaceous milk substitutes. Many of the calves, especially the bull calves, are killed, thus leaving all the milk for human use. When cows cease to yield sufficient milk they too are slaughtered. Milch cows are commonly kept in unhealthy houses, deprived of exercise and pure air, crowded together, with filthy evil smelling floors reeking with their excrements, tended by uncleanly people. With no exercise and a rich stimulating diet they produce more milk; but it is no matter for surprise that tuberculosis is common amongst them. When the lesions of tubercle (consumption) are localised and not excessive, the rest of the carcase is passed by veterinary surgeons as fit for food; were it otherwise, enormous quantities of meat would be destroyed. As butcher's meat is seldom officially inspected, but a very small part is judged by the butchers as too bad for food. In mitigation it may be said that poultry lead a happy existence and their death is, or should be, quickly produced with but little pain, probably less pain than if left to die from natural causes. The same cannot be said of cattle and sheep when the time arrives for their transport to the slaughter man's. It is argued by vegetarians who take milk and animal products that they are not responsible for the death of the animals, as they do not eat their flesh. As vegetarians profit by conditions in which the slaughtering of the animals is a part, they cannot be altogether exonerated. Cow's milk is prone to absorb bad odours, and it forms a most suitable breeding or nutrient medium for most species of bacteria which may accidentally get therein. By means of milk many epidemics have been spread, of scarlet fever, diphtheria, cholera, and typhoid. Occasionally milk contains tubercle bacilli from the cows themselves. By boiling, all bacteria, except a few which may be left out of consideration, are destroyed. Such a temperature, however, renders the milk less digestible and wholesome for infants. By heating to 160° F. or 170° F. for a few minutes, such pathogenic germs as are at all likely to be in milk (tubercle, typhoid, diphtheria, &c.) are killed, and the value of the milk is but little affected: this is called Pasteurising. It was until quite recently a common practice to add boric acid, formaldehyde and other preservatives; this has injured the vitality and caused the death of many infants. They have not yet gone quite out of use.

For infants the only satisfactory food is that of a healthy mother. On account of physical defects in the mother, or often for merely selfish reasons, the infant is deprived of its natural food. Many attempts have been made to bring cow's milk to approximately the same composition as human milk. It can be done by adding water, milk sugar and cream of known composition, in certain proportions. Great difficulties are met with when this is put into practice. The simplest method is that of Professor Soxhlet. The proper quantity of milk sugar is added, but instead of adding the right quantity of cream or fat—a very difficult thing to do—the equivalent quantity of extra milk sugar is used. Although not theoretically satisfactory, in practice it answers very well. We have found it to agree very well with infants. To cow's milk of pure average quality, add half its volume of water containing 12.3 per cent. of milk sugar; or, what amounts to the same thing, to a pint of cow's milk add one and a quarter ounce of milk sugar and half-a-pint of water. It is preferable to Pasteurise by placing the bottle of milk in a vessel of water. This water is to be heated until the milk shows a temperature of about 75° C. or 165° F., but must not exceed 80° C. or a change in the albumen of the milk takes place which affects its digestibility. Keep at this temperature for about ten minutes. If not required at once, a plug of cotton wool should be placed in the neck of the bottle, and it should be kept in a cold place until required. Professor Soxhlet does not advise the addition of lime water. The proteids are not of the same composition as in human milk (the calf being a ruminating animal)—and it is a common plan to add water or barley water to milk until it is so watered down that it cannot curdle into tough curds. An infant has thus either to distend its stomach with a large quantity of watery nourishment, or else to get insufficient food. Sometimes it is necessary to peptonise the milk a little. At the Leipzig infants hospital, and also the Hygienic Institute, they give to infants, up to 9 months old, Prof. Soxhlet's mixture, except that an equal volume of water is added to the milk. Milk, cheese, and especially hen's eggs contain a very large proportion of proteid. When added to food poor in proteid they improve its nutritive quality. It has often been said, and with truth, that some vegetarians by the profuse use of animal products, consume as much, or even more proteid of animal origin than the average person who includes flesh food in his dietary. An excess of proteid from these sources is less injurious as eggs contain no purins, and milk but a very small quantity. In support of the use of animal products, it may be said that we have become so fond of animal foods and stimulating drinks, that the use of milk, butter, cheese and eggs renders the transition to a dietary derived from the vegetable kingdom much easier. By means of these, cooked dishes can be produced which approach and sometimes can scarcely be distinguished from those of cooked flesh.

In the present state of society, when really good vegetarian fare is difficult to procure away from home, eggs, cheese, and milk are a great convenience.

Digestion.—The digestive juices contain certain unorganised ferments, which produce chemical changes in the food. If the food is solid, it has to be liquefied. Even if already liquid it has generally to undergo a chemical change before being fitted for absorption into the body. The alimentary canal is a tubular passage which is first expanded into the mouth, and later into the stomach. As the food passes down, it is acted upon by several digestive juices, and in the small intestine the nutritive matter is absorbed, whilst the residue passes away.

The saliva is the first digestive juice. It is alkaline and contains a ferment called ptyalin. This acts energetically on the cooked and gelatinous starch, and slowly on the raw starch. Starch is quite insoluble in water, but the first product of salivary digestion is a less complex substance called soluble-starch. When time is allowed for the action to be completed, the starch is converted into one of the sugars called maltose. In infants this property of acting on starch does not appear in effective degree until the sixth or seventh month, and starch should not be given before that time. Only a small quantity should be provided before the twelfth month, when it may be gradually increased. Dr. Sims Wallace has suggested that the eruption of the lower incisors from the seventh to the eighth month, was for the purpose of enabling the infant—in the pre-cooking stage of man's existence—to pierce the outer covering of fruits so as to permit his extracting the soluble contents by suction; and accordingly when these teeth are cut we may allow the child to bite at such vegetable substances as apples, oranges, and sugar cane. Dr. Harry Campbell says that starch should be given to the young, "not as is the custom, as liquid or pap, but in a form compelling vigorous mastication, for it is certain that early man, from the time he emerged from the ape till he discovered how to cook his vegetable food, obtained practically all his starch in such a form. If it is given as liquid or pap it will pass down as starch into the stomach, to setup disturbance in that organ; while if it is administered in a form which obliges the child to chew it properly, not only will the jaws, the teeth, and the gums obtain the exercise which they crave, and without which they cannot develop normally, but the starch will be thoroughly insalivated that much of it will be converted within the mouth into maltose. Hard well baked crusts constitute a convenient form in which to administer starch to children. A piece of crust may be put in the oven and rebaked, and spread with butter. Later, we may give hard plain biscuits." Dr. Campbell continues, that he does not say that starch in the pappy form, or as porridge, should find no place whatever in man's dietary at the present day, but we should arrange that a large proportion of our food is in a form inviting mastication.

The teeth perform the very important function of breaking down our food and enabling it to be intimately incorporated with the saliva and afterwards with the digestive juices. The Anglo-Saxon race shows a greater tendency to degeneracy in the teeth than do other races; the teeth of the present generation are less perfect than those of previous generations. A dentist writes (*Lancet*, 1903-2, p. 1054) "I have had the opportunity of examining the teeth of many natives in their more or less uncivilised state, from the Red Indians of North America, the negroes of Africa, to the more civilised Chinese, Japanese, and Indians of the East, and I have usually found them possessed of sound teeth, but so soon as they come under the influence of civilised life in Washington, Montreal, London, Paris and other cities, their teeth begin to degenerate, though their general health may remain good." In a long article on mastication in the *Lancet* (1903-2, p. 84) from which we have already quoted, Dr. Harry Campbell gives as the effect of thorough and efficient mastication, that it increases the amount of alkaline saliva passing into the stomach, and prolongs the period of starch digestion within that organ. That it influences the stomach reflexly by promoting the flow of gastric juice. That the frequent use of the jaws and the tongue, during the period of growth, cause the jaws to expand. If the jaws are not adequately exercised during this period, owing to the use of soft food, they do not reach their normal size, the teeth are overcrowded, do not develop fully, and are prone to decay. The effect of vigorous mastication is to stimulate the circulation in the tooth pulp, which promotes nutrition and maintains a firm dental setting. Dr. Campbell writes: "I am perfectly at one with Dr. Wallace, in believing that the removal of the fibrous portion of food is the main cause of the prevalence of caries among moderns."

When the food reaches the stomach, gastric juice is secreted. This juice contains a ferment called pepsin and hydrochloric acid. Pepsin is only active in an acid media. Starch digestion proceeds in the stomach to such a time—stated as from 15 to 30 minutes—when the acid gastric juice has been poured out in sufficient quantity to neutralise the alkalinity of the saliva. The gastric juice acts upon the proteids only. After a time the liquefied contents of the stomach are passed into the first portion of the small intestine, called the duodenum. Here it meets with the pancreatic juice, which like the gastric juice attacks proteids, but even more energetically, and only in an alkaline media. The proteolitic ferment is called trypsin. The pancreatic, the most important of the digestive fluids, contains other ferments; one called amylopsin, takes up the digestion of any remaining or imperfectly converted starch left from the salivary digestion. Amylopsin is much more powerful and rapid than the ptyalin of the saliva, especially on uncooked starch. Its absence from the pancreatic juice of infants is an indication that starch should not be given them. Another ferment, stearopsin, emulsifies fats. The bile is alkaline and assists the pancreatic juice in neutralising the acid mixture that leaves the stomach; it also assists the absorption of fats. The digestion of proteids is not completed in the stomach. There are some who look upon the stomach as chiefly of use as a receptacle for the large mass of food, which is too quickly eaten to be passed at once into the intestines; the food being gradually expelled from the stomach, in such quantities as the duodenal digestion can adequately treat. A frequently used table, showing the time required for the digestion of various foods in the stomach, is of little practical value. There is ample provision for the digestion of food, there is a duplication of ferments for the proteids and starch. In health, the ferments are not only very active, but are secreted in ample quantities. The digestive or unorganised ferments must not be confused with the organised ferments such as yeast. The latter are living vegetable cells, capable of indefinite multiplication. The former are soluble bodies, and though capable of transforming or digesting some thousands of times their mass of food, their power in this direction is restricted within definite limits. Another and preferable name for them is enzymes.

The action of saliva on starch is powerfully retarded by tea, this is due to the tannin. Coffee and cocoa are without effect. Tea infused for two minutes only, was not found to have sensibly less restraining effect than when infused for thirty minutes. On peptic digestion both tea and coffee had a powerful retarding effect. When of equal strength cocoa was nearly as bad, but as it is usually taken much weaker, its inhibitory effect is of little consequence.

Bacteria are minute vegetable organisms, which exist in the dust of the air, in water and almost everywhere on or near the surface of the earth. They are consequently taken in with our food. They exist in the mouth; those in carious teeth are often sufficient to injuriously affect digestion and health. The healthy gastric juice is to a great degree antiseptic, but few bacteria being able to endure its acidity. When the residue of the food reaches the large intestine, bacteria are found in very great numbers. The warmth of the body is highly favourable to their growth. They cause the food and intestinal *debris* to assume its fæcal character. Should the mass be retained, the bacterial poisons accumutate and being absorbed into the body produce headaches, exhaustion, neurasthenia and other complaints. Proteid matter, the products of its decomposition and nitrogenous matter generally, are especially the food of bacteria; this is shown in the offensiveness of the fæces of the carnivora, notwithstanding their short intestines, compared with that of the herbivora. Also in the difference of the fæces of the dog when fed on flesh and on a nearly vegetable diet. On a rich proteid diet, especially if it consists largely of flesh, the bacterial products in the intestines are greater than on a vegetable diet. On the latter such a disease as appendicitis is rare. Professor Elie Metchnikoff, of the Pasteur Institute, thinks that man's voluminous and highly developed large intestine fulfils no useful purpose, and on account of its breeding a very copious and varied bacterial flora, could with advantage be dispensed with. He also has said that man, who could support himself on food easily digestible, has a small intestine which is disproportionately fully developed. Instead of having between 18 and 21 feet of small intestine, man might do with one-third of that length. According to him, there is a disharmony of our food and our digestive system. Referring to such views, and the desire of some surgeons to remove the vermiform appendix and portions of the intestines upon too little provocation, Sir W. Macewin, M.D., F.R.S. (*B. Medical Jrn.*, 1904, 2 p. 874) says:—"Is this human body of ours so badly constructed that it contains so many useless parts and requires so much tinkering? Possibly I may be out of fashion with the times, as I cannot find such imperfections in the normal human body as are alleged. On the contrary, the more one looks into the human body and sees it work, the better one understands it and the more one is struck with the wondrous utility, beauty, and harmony of all its parts." Our food we can change, but not our organs-except by a dangerous surgical operations. Our teeth with our complex and very long intestines are adapted for fibrous, bulky and solid food. On such food mankind has lived for an immense period of time. It is true that there are several theoretical advantages in cooked vegetable foods; but unfortunately there is a want of conformity with our digestive organs. If a flesh diet is taken, the incongruity is greater. Concentrated food causes constipation. An active man, leading an out-of-door life, can take unsuitable food with little or no apparent inconvenience, the movements of his body favouring intestinal action; whilst the same food to a sedentary person will prove distinctly injurious.

Some persons have such a vigorous digestion that they can consume almost any food, even that which is obviously unsuitable; not only bad in kind but excessive in quantity. Other persons have to be very careful. Many have boasted that they can take of what they call the good things of life to their full, without bad effect. We know of such men who have been much esteemed for their joviality and good nature, but who have broken down in what should have been a hearty and useful middle life. There are others who were poorly equipped for the battle of life, with indifferent constitutions, never having had the buoyancy and overflowing of animal spirits; but who, by conserving such strength as they had, have outlived all their more healthy but less careful comrades. The errors of the parents are often most evident in the children or grandchildren. There are many persons who cannot eat of some particular food, although it may be quite wholesome to others. Sometimes it is a psychological rather than a physiological disability, which may he overcome by an effort of the will. At other times it seems to have no connection with the imagination, although it is not always possible to give a sound reason for it. In the main, of course, there are principles of dietetics applicable to all alike, but in regard to details, everyone should make rules for himself, according to his experience. When there appears no real reason for an idiosyncrasy, a little humouring of our taste and digestion will often overcome it, to our advantage. It is generally those of delicate constitution who are most sensitive. Some cannot eat oatmeal except in small quantity. Olive and other vegetable oils, even when of good quality cannot be taken by many people, whilst others find them quite as wholesome, or even better than butter. Vegetarians can generally detect lard in pastry both by its taste and its after effects, although those accustomed to this fat do not object to it. It is also surprising how some individual's tastes and habits will vary at different periods of their lives.

One form of dyspepsia is due to undigested starch remaining in the stomach and causing an excessive secretion of hydrochloric acid. As long as proteid food is present, the pepsin and acid expend themselves on it, and are removed together. The undigested starch continues to stimulate gastric secretion, and the acid residuum causes pain, heartburn and flatulence. If there be also any butyric acid, or some other fatty acid, derived from milk, butter, cheese, &c., there will be acid eructations. For this form of indigestion there are several methods of treatment. First; the very thorough cooking of all starchy food, and it is an advantage to take a little good extract of malt, either at the time of eating or directly afterwards. The diastase of the malt has the same action on starch as the ptyalin in the saliva. It is better, scientifically, to have the farinaceous food at about 130° F. (as hot as the mouth can bear will do), and then to add malt extract. On keeping the mixture warm, from a few minutes to half an hour or more, the starch is digested and rendered soluble. Such food is not very pleasant to take. The food known as Grape Nuts has been treated in a similar manner. The use of malt extract, however, seems a clumsy substitute for salivary digestion. Second; the eating of starch in the form of hard and dry biscuits, crusts and other hard food, which demand thorough mastication and insalivation, and the keeping in the mouth for a long while, during which the saliva has time to act. This is the best plan. Third; the taking of sodium bicarbonate towards the end of the period of digestion, in order to neutralise the acid in the stomach. This gives relief, but does not cure, as the dose has to be repeated after each meal; in course of time the quantity of soda has sometimes to be increased to an alarming extent. Fourth; the abstention from starchy foods and the substitution of an exclusive flesh dietary. In the "Salisbury" treatment, raw minced beef is given. This method often gives immediate relief, but its ultimate effect on the kidneys and other organs is very bad.

No hard and fast rule can be laid down as to the number of meals into which the daily amount of food required should be divided. The stomach appears to work to the best advantage when it is full, or nearly so, and the appetite is appeased. Three approximately equal meals seems to be a convenient division. Dr. Dewey and his followers advise only two meals a day, and it seems incontestable that many persons find the plan advantageous. These are generally adults with weak digestions, or elderly persons who, on account of their age and the sluggish action of their assimilative functions, require comparatively little food. Children, on account of their vigorous vitality, rapid growth and hearty appetites, ought not to be restricted to this number. Persons who have got into the pernicious habit of greatly over-eating, and whose stomachs have become distended and unusually large, sometimes find it easier to restrict their daily food to a healthy quantity by taking only two meals. The general objections against two meals are that either two little food is taken, or the ingestion of such a large quantity is bad for the stomach and causes it to press on the adjacent viscera. The large quantity of blood and nerve force drawn to the over-distended stomach, depletes the brain and nervous system, causing drowsiness and incapacity for mental and physical work. The carnivora, whose opportunity for obtaining food—unlike the herbivora—is irregular and often at long intervals, gorge themselves upon opportunity and are in the habit of sleeping after a meal. The frugivora and herbivora, however, are alert and ready to fly from their enemies should such appear. The conveying of so much nourishment to the liver and blood stream at one time, is probably a greater tax on them. A light lunch between the usual full meals has nothing to recommend it. The stomach is burdened to little purpose, often before it has finished with one meal another is imposed upon it, no time being left for recuperation.

Dietaries.—The best proportions of proteids, carbo-hydrates and fats required for the nourishment of the body has not yet been conclusively decided. The common plan is to average the dietary of large bodies of persons, particualrly of soldiers and prisoners. These dietaries have been adjusted empirically (the earlier ones at least), and are generally considered as satisfactory. They are chiefly of English and German origin. Another method is to laboriously analyse the injesta or food consumed and compare it with the dejecta or excretions, until a quantity and kind of food is found which is just sufficient to keep the body in equilibrium. This latter plan is the best, but to be quite satisfactory must be tried on a large number of suitable persons under varying conditions, both of quantity and kind of food. Nearly all the experiments have been made on persons accustomed to a stimulating dietary: their usual food has included a considerable quantity of flesh and alcoholic drinks. Sufficient attention has not been paid to the dietaries of the more abstemious races who partake of little if any flesh food. The standard daily dietary for a man of average weight, doing a moderate amount of work, is variously stated by the

best authorities as proteids from 100 to 130 grammes, fat 35 to 125 grammes, and carbo-hydrates 450 to 550 grammes. There is a surprising difference of opinion on the amount of fat, but those who give least fat give the largest quantity of carbo-hydrate and *vice-versa*. Dr. R. Hutchison in "Food and Dietetics," sums up the quantities given by the highest authorities as follows:
—-

Proteid	125 g. (4.4 oz.) x 4.1 =	512 cal. = 20 g. N,	62 C
Carbo-hydrate	500 g. (17.6 oz.) 4.1	2050	200
Fat	50 g. (1.8 oz.) 9.3	465	38
	675 g. (23.8 oz.)	3027 Total 20 g. N,	300 C

The nutrient ratio is 1 : 4.9. For scientific purposes, metrical weights and measures are used, instead of the inconvenient English grains, ounces, pounds, &c. (1 gramme = 15.43 grains; 1 ounce avoirdupois = 437.5 grains = 28.35 grammes). A calorie is a measure of the power of a food in generating heat and muscular energy (these two being convertible).

The calories used in food tables are kilo-calories, representing the amount of heat which would raise a kilogramme (1000 grammes) of water 1° Centigrade. This is the same as raising 1 pound weight 4° Fahrenheit. According to the table given, 125 grammes of dry proteid are required per day; this contains 20 grammes of nitrogen and 62 of carbon. When thoroughly consumed or utilised in the body, the heat or its equivalent in muscular work equals 512 kilo-calories. Proteids have, of course, an additional value as tissue formers. The factors used here, of 4.1 and 9.3, are those commonly employed; but the latest and most reliable research, taking account only of that part of the food which is actually available in the body, gives for proteid and carbo-hydrate 4 calories, and for fat 8.9 calories.

Fat has a higher food value than the carbo-hydrates, as 4.1 : 9.3 = 2.27 or 4.0 : 89 = 2.225, according to whether the old or new factors are used. In the table of analyses 2.225 was used. The standard dietary for a woman, or of a boy 14 to 16 years of age, is given as equivalent to eight-tenths that of a man; a child of 10 to 13 six-tenths; of 2 to 5 four-tenths. A man doing hard work requires one-tenth more. The following table gives three standard dietaries, and a few actual ones, in grammes per day. The food of persons in easy circumstances, and of working men in the receipt of good wages, approximate to the standard dietaries, except that the fat is higher and the carbo-hydrates proportionately less. This is due to an abundance of animal food. It was thought unnecessary to give them in detail:—

	Pr't.	Fat.	C'r'b.	Cal.	N. R.
Hutchison : Man, moderate muscular work	125	50	500	3027	4·9
Atwater : ,, ,, ,, ,,	125	...	...	3400	6·2
Voit : ,, ,, ,, ,,	118	56	500	2965	5·5
Atwater : Woman, light to moderate muscular work, or Man without muscular exercise	90	...	...	2450	6·1
Football teams, Connecticut and California, U.S.	226	354	634	6590	6·6
Russian peasants	129	33	589	3165	5·4
Negro families—Alabama and Virginia	86	145	440	3395	9·3
Labourers—Lombardy (diet, mostly vegetable)	82	40	362	2192	5·5
Japanese, on vegetable diet (a)	71	12	396	2026	6·0
Trappist monk, in Cloisters—vegetable diet	68	11	469	2304	7·3
Java village—Columbia Exposition, 1893	66	19	254	1450	4·7
Sewing girl—London (3/9 per week)	53	33	316	1820	7·3
German vegetarians	54	22	573	2775	11·6
German labourers' family (poor circumstances)	52	32	287	1640	7·2
Dr. T. R. A.—wheatmeal bread and water only (b)	82	8·5	470	2342	6·0
Man—3 years' exclusively vegetable diet (c)	54	22	557	2710	11·2
Thomas Wood, the miller of Billericay (d)	55	5·7	313	1560	6·0

Dr. Alexander Haig considers that 88 grammes of proteid is required by a man leading a decidedly active life.

NOTES.—(a) The Japanese are of small stature and weight.

(b) One of a series of experiments by A.W. Blyth, 1888. 1½ lbs. of wheatmeal per day was required for equilibrium; sedentary occupation, with a daily walk of six miles.

(*c*) See "A Text Book of Physiology," by M. Foster, 5th edition, part ii., p. 839; the diet was bread, fruit and oil. The man was in apparently good health and stationary weight; only 59 per cent. of the proteids were digested, leaving the small quantity of 32 grammes available for real use. In commenting upon this, Professor Foster writes:—"We cannot authoritatively say that such a reduction is necessarily an evil; for our knowledge will not at present permit us to make an authoritative exact statement as to the extent to which the proteid may be reduced without disadvantage to the body, when accompanied by adequate provision of the other elements of food; and this statement holds good whether the body be undertaking a small or large amount of labour."

(*d*) The Miller of Billericay's case is quoted by Dr. Carpenter, and also by Dr. Pavy. It was reported to the College of Physicians in 1767 by Sir George Baker. A remarkable degree of vigour is said to have been sustained for upwards of eighteen years on no other nutriment than 16 oz. of flour, made into a pudding with water, no other liquid of any kind being taken.

A striking instance of abstemiousness is that of Cornaro, a Venetian nobleman, who died in the year 1566 at the age of 98. Up to the age of 40 he spent a life of indulgence, eating and drinking to excess. At this time, having been endowed with a feeble constitution, he was suffering from dyspepsia, gout, and an almost continual slow fever, with an intolerable thirst continually hanging upon him. The skill of the best physicians of Italy was unavailing. At length he completely changed his habits of diet, and made a complete recovery. At the age of 83 he wrote a treatise on a "Sure and certain method of attaining a long and healthful life." He says, what with bread, meat, the yolk of an egg and soup, I ate as much as weighed 12 ozs., neither more nor less. I drank 14 oz. of wine. When 78 he was persuaded to increase his food by the addition of 2 oz. per day, and this nearly proved fatal. He writes that, instead of old age being one of weakness, infirmity and misery, I find myself to be in the most pleasant and delightful stage of life. At 83 I am always merry, maintaining a happy peace in my own mind. A sober life has preserved me in that sprightliness of thought and gaiety of humour. My teeth are all as sound as in my youth. He was able to take moderate exercise in riding and walking at that age. He was very passionate and hasty in his youth. He wrote other treatises up to the age of 95.

Kumagara, Lapicque and Breis-acher, have, as the result of their experiments, reduced the quantity of proteid required per 24 hours to 45 grammes. T.

Hirschfeld states, as the conclusion of his research, that it is possible for a healthy man (in one case for 15 days and in another for 10 days) to maintain nitrogenous balance on from 30 to 40 grammes of proteid per day. Labbé and Morchoisne (Comptes Rendus, 30th May, 1904, p. 1365) made a dieting experiment during 38 days, upon one of themselves. The proteid was derived exclusively from vegetable food. The food consisted of bread, lentils, haricots, potatoes, carrots, chestnuts, endives, apples, oranges, preserves, sugar, starch, butter, chocolate and wine. At the commencement, the day's food contained 14.1 grammes of nitrogen = 89.3 proteid, which was gradually diminished. On the 7th day 11.6 g. N. = 73.5 g. proteid was reached; during this time less N. was eliminated, indicating that the proteid food was in excess of that required for the wear and tear of the body. As the quantity of nitrogenous food was diminished almost daily, the N. eliminated was found to diminish also. This latter was in slight excess of that absorbed; but when a day or two's time was allowed, without further reduction in the food, the body tended to adjust itself to the dimished supply, and there was an approximation of income and expenditure. The smallest quantity of food was reached on the 32nd day with 1.06 N. = 6.7 proteid, which was obviously too little, as 2.19 N. = 13.9 proteid was eliminated. On the 21st day 4.12 N. = 26 proteid was injested, and 4.05 N. was eliminated. The inference drawn from the research is that about 26 grammes of proteid per day was sufficient. The weight of the body remained practically constant throughout, and the subject did not suffer inconvenience. Of course the full amount of calories was kept up; as each succeeding quantity of the proteid was left off, it was replaced by a proper quantity of non-nitrogenous food. These experiments were carried out in the usual approved scientific manner. It may, however, be urged against any generalised and positive conclusions as to the minimum quantity of proteid required for the body, being drawn from such experiments, that the period covered by them was much too short. A prolonged trial might have revealed some obscure physiological derangement. We are quite justified in concluding that the usual, so-called "standard dietaries" contain an unnecessarily large proportion of proteid. In some practical dietaries, 50 grammes and under have seemed enough; but for the ordinary adult man, who has been accustomed to an abundance of proteid, and whose ancestors have also, it is probably advisable not to take less than 70 or 80 grammes per day (2½ to 3 ounces). If it is desired to try less, the diminution should be very gradual, and a watch should be kept for any lessening of strength.

Some comments may now be made upon the table of dietaries. That of the London sewing girl contained 53 grammes of proteid, which should have been ample, according to some of the authorities we have given; yet she was badly nourished. The food was doubtless of bad quality, and it appears deficient in carbo-hydrates; this latter is shown by the low number of calories. The long hours and unhealthy conditions of work, and not a deficiency of food constituents, is probably the cause of the bad health of such persons. There is no reason to think the proteid insufficient, although some persons have said as much. We have no particulars of the German vegetarians, but the calories appear satisfactory. In the poor German labourer's family the calories are too low. In Dr. T.R. Allinson's experiment on a wheatmeal dietary, it will not do to assume that less than 82 grammes of proteid would have been insufficient. It is probable that a smaller quantity of proteid would have been enough if the fat and carbohydrates had been increased. The calories are below the usual standard. In the succeeding example the calories are considerably higher, being not far from the usual standard, yet 54 grammes of proteid sufficed. It is a common error to place an undue value on the proteids to the extent of overlooking the other constituents. Dr. Alexander Haig in "Diet and Food," p. 8, cites the case of a boy aged 10, fed on 2¼ pints of milk per day. The boy lost weight, and Dr. Haig is of opinion that the quantity of milk was very deficient in proteid; more than twice as much being required. 2¼ pints of milk contain about 45 grammes of proteid, whereas, according to the usual figures (125 x 6/10) a boy of this age requires 75 g. This quantity of 45 g. is however, higher, allowing for the boy's age, than that in several of the dietaries we have given in our table. A little consideration will show that Dr. Haig has overlooked the serious deficiency of the milk in the other constituents, which accounts for the boy's loss of weight. The quantity of milk contains only about 160 g. of total solid matter, whilst 400 g. is the necessary quantity. Milk is too rich in proteid matter to form, with advantage, the sole food of a human being. Human milk contains much less in proportion to the other constituents.

The old doctrine enunciated by Justus von Liebig was that proteid matter is the principal source of muscular energy or strength. He afterwards discovered and acknowledged his error, and the subject has since been thoroughly investigated. The makers of meat extracts and other foods, either from their own ignorance of modern research or their wish to take advantage of the lack of knowledge and prejudice of the public, call proteid matter alone nourishment. The carbo-hydrates and fats are equally entitled to be called nourishment.

Our reason for devoting so much space to the consideration of the quantity of proteid matter required, is that in the opinion of many eminent writers it is the crux of vegetarianism. They have stated that it is impossible to obtain sufficient from vegetable foods alone, without consuming an excessive quantity of carbo-hydrates. We will summarise the argument as given in Kirke's Physiology, as edited by Morrant Baker, a standard work, and which is repeated in Furneaux's "Animal Physiology," a book which is much used in elementary science schools: "The daily waste from the system amounts to, carbon 4,500 grains (or 300 grammes), and nitrogen, 300 grains (or 20 grammes). Now let us suppose a person to feed on bread only. In order to obtain the necessary quantity of nitrogen to repair this waste he would have to eat nearly 4¼ lbs. daily.... He would be compelled to take about double the quantity of carbon required in order to obtain the necessary weight of nitrogen.... Next, let us suppose that he feeds on lean meat only. Then, in order to obtain the necessary quantity of carbon, he must eat no less than 6½ lbs. daily.... In this case we notice a similar waste of nitrogen, the removal of which would give an undue amount of work to the organs concerned.... But it is possible to take such a mixed diet of bread and meat as will supply all the requirements of the system, and at the same time yield but little waste material." (These extracts are from Furneaux, the next is from Kirke. The figures and argument is the same in each, but we have chosen those sentences for quotation which are the briefest and most suitable; certain calculations being omitted.) "A combination of bread and meat would supply much more economically what was necessary ... so that ¾ lbs. of meat, and less than 2 lbs. of bread would supply all the needful carbon and nitrogen with but little waste. From these facts it will be plain that a mixed diet is the best and most economical food for man; and the result of experience entirely coincides with what might have been anticipated on theoretical grounds only." Professor Huxley, in his "Elementary Physiology" uses almost the same figures and argument.

The adoption of this high proteid or nitrogen figure would lead to some ridiculous conclusions. One writer states that 18 eggs would contain sufficient flesh forming substance for a day's ration, but a very much larger quantity would be required to supply enough carbon. On the other hand, Professor Church says that, no less than 70 lbs. of pears would have to be eaten per day, to supply the necessary quantity of nitrogen; although the carbon would be in excess. The curious may calculate the proper quantity of each that would make a theoretically perfect dietary. People are apt to assume that what they themselves eat, or what their class, race, or nation eat, is the proper and necessary diet; at least as far as the elementary constituents and quantities are concerned. The error is in attempting to make a vegetarian diet, however contrary to common sense and the experience of the greater part of the earth's inhabitants, agree in composition with the ordinary lavish flesh dietary of the well-to-do European. It is significant that John Bull is caricatured with a large abdomen and a coarse, ruddy, if not inflamed face, indicative of his hearty dining on flesh, coarse food and alcoholic drinks. An unhealthy short lived individual. Even if we accept a high proportion of proteid, it is possible to combine purely vegetable foods so as to give the required quantity of the various constituents, without a superfluity of the carbo-hydrates. In "Food Grains of India," Professor A.H. Church shows by elaborate analyses and dietary tables, how this can be accomplished by various combinations of cereals, pulses, etc. He takes Forster and Voit's standard of 282 grains of nitrogen and 5,060 grains of carbon, with a suitable deduction for the smaller weight of the Indians. In his examples of daily rations he gives from 5 to 9 ounces of various beans, balanced by the addition of the proper quantity of rice —4 to 16 ounces, and a little oil. Such a large quantity of pulse appears to us excessive, and would cause discomfort to most persons. We much doubt whether those Indians who are strict vegetarians could consume such quantities.

Some valuable investigations were made on the diet of a family of fruitarians, at the Californian Agricultural Experimental Station, July, 1900, by Professor M.E. Jaffa (bulletin 107). The proportion of food, both proteid and carbo-hydrate used was surprisingly small. The research is particularly important, as the diet was not an experimental one, tried during a short period only; but that to which the family were accustomed. The family consisted of two women and three children; they had all been fruitarians for five to seven years, and made no change in their dietary during the experiment. They only had two meals a day, the food being eaten uncooked. The quantities of all the foods and other particulars are detailed in the bulletin. The first meal was at 10-30 a.m., and always consisted of nuts followed by fruits. The other meal was about 5 p.m., when they usually ate no nuts, substituting olive oil and honey. The nuts used were almonds, Brazil, pine, pignolias and walnuts; the fresh fruits were apples, apricots, bananas, figs, grapes, oranges, peaches and pears. Other foods were dates, raisins, pickled olives, olive oil and honey. One person (b) ate a little celery and tomatoes, and another (c) a little cereal food. In the following table are given the average daily quantities of the food constituents in grammes:—

Proteids, fat, carbo-hydrate, crude fibre, value in calories and nutrient ratio. The crude fibre is classed as a carbo-hydrate and included in the calorie value, and also in calculating the nutrient ratio.

	Pro.	Fat.	C'r'b.	Fibre.	Cal.	N. R.
Woman, age 33, weight 90 lbs. (a)	33	59	110	40	1300	8·6
Woman ,, 30 ,, 104 ,, (b)	25	57	72	27	1040	9·1
Girl ,, 13 ,, 75½ ,, (c)	26	52	111	46	1235	10·5
Boy ,, 9 ,, 43 ,, (d)	27	56	102	50	1255	10·3
Girl ,, 6 ,, 30½ ,, (e)	24	58	97	37	1190	11·1
Girl ,, 7 ,, 34 ,, (ee)	40	72	126	8	1385	7·4

The last research extended over ten days; the period during which each of the other subjects was under observation was from 20 to 28 days.

(a) The tentative standard for a woman at light work calls for 90 grammes of proteids and 2,500 calories; it is thus seen that the quantity of food eaten was far below that usually stated as being necessary. The subject, however, was a very small woman, 5 feet in height, taking almost no physical exercise. She believed, as do fruitarians generally, that people need far less raw than cooked food. (b) The food eaten was even less in quantity than in the previous dietary. One reason for this was the fact that the subject was, for part of the time at least, under great mental strain, and did not have her usual appetite. Even this small amount of food, judging by her appearance and manner, seemed sufficient for her needs, enabling her to do her customary housework and take care of her two nieces and nephew, the subjects of the other experiments. (c) This girl was given cereals and vegetables when she craved them, but her aunt says she never looks nor feels so well when she has much starchy food, and returns to her next meal of uncooked food with an increased appreciation of its superiority. The commonly accepted dietary standard for a child 13 years old and of average activity, is not far from 90 grammes of proteids and 2,450 calories, yet the girl had all the appearance of being well fed and in excellent health and spirits. (d) During the 22 days of experiment, there was an increase in weight of 2 pounds, due to the fact that the family had been in straitened circumstances, and the food provided was more abundant during the study. (e) The subject had been very delicate as a baby. She was very small for her age, being 10 pounds under the average weight, and 7 inches less than the average height. It is interesting to note that her only gain in weight during the past year was made during this dietary and the one immediately following. This was due to her being urged to eat all she wanted, of what she most preferred, as the food was provided by those making the study. The proteid is less than the tentative standard for a child of 1 to 2 years old, but the subject appeared perfectly well and was exceedingly active. She impressed one as being a healthy child, but looked younger than her age. (*ee*) The subject is the same as in the previous experiment (*e*), but after an interval of 8 months, her seventh birthday occurred during the time.

Professor Jaffa, who made the investigation, says:—"It would appear that all the subjects were decidedly under-nourished, even making allowance for their light weight. But when we consider that the two adults have lived upon this diet for seven years, and think they are in better health and capable of more work than they ever were before, we hesitate to pronounce judgment. The three children had the appearance of health and strength. They ran and jumped and played all day like ordinary healthy children, and were said to be unusually free from colds and other complaints common to childhood. The youngest child, and the only one who has lived as a fruitarian almost from infancy was certainly undeveloped. She looked fully two years younger than she was. Still, there are so many children who are below the average in development, whose dietaries conform to the ordinary standards, that it would be unfair to draw any conclusions until many more such investigations are made."

The research shows that not only is there need of a revision of the "standard" quantity of proteids, but also of the carbo-hydrates and fats. It is generally said by those who have no practical experience amongst vegetarians, that the latter require a much larger quantity of food than do those who include flesh. The truth is that vegetarians eat less, often much less. It is a common experience that vegetable food has a more staying power, and a much longer period can be allowed between meals, without the inconvenience that a flesh-eater, especially a flesh and alcohol consumer, suffers. This is due, in part at least, to its less stimulating character and its slower digestion. This fact has been shown by the success of vegetarians in feats of strength and endurance, and especially in the comparatively fresh condition in which they have finished long walking, cycling, tennis, and other matches. Those who attempt to prolong their powers of endurance by flesh extracts and stimulating foods and drinks, usually finish in a very exhausted condition. The superior endurance and recovery from wounds, when compared with our English soldiers, of simple feeding men, such as the Zulus, Turks and Japanese, has often been remarked. It is often said that vegetable food, as it contains more fibre and is slower of digestion, taxes the bodily organs more. If we attempted to eat uncooked, the more fibrous vegetables, the grains, and unripe fruit, it would be quite true, but it is not so of the ordinary food of vegetarians. A slowness of digestion does not necessarily imply a greater strain on the system. As vegetables, in particular, are for the longest period of time in the intestines, and undergo the greater part of their digestion there, a gentle and slow process of digestion in that organ may be more thorough. It may also entail less expenditure of nervous energy than if the food had been of such a stimulating character, as to be hurried along the digestive tract. Digestion is for the most part a chemical process. If the food is of right kind and quantity, thoroughly masticated, assisted if necessary by cookery, and the digestive ferments are normal, digestion proceeds without any sensible expenditure or energy or consciousness of its accomplishment. There is nothing improbable in a flesh-eater requiring more food than a simple living vegetarian. His food contains more proteid, and excrementitious matter or extractives; these stimulate the digestive organs and overtax the excretory ones. Generally, he is fond of condiments, salt, and elaborate cooking, often also of alcohol; if a man, probably of tobacco. He lives, as it were, at high pressure.

There are on record certain experiments which appear to indicate the necessity of a large proportion of proteid, especially when the diet has been of vegetable origin. These experiments are inconclusive, because the subject has been accustomed to an ordinary flesh diet, perhaps also to alcoholic drinks. The change to a comparatively non-stimulating diet cannot be made, and the digestive organs expected to adapt themselves in a few days. Perhaps not even a month or a year would suffice, for some people, and yet that same diet would suit others. In some experiments the food has not been appetising, the subject has even taken it with reluctance or even loathing; an excess of some food has been eaten which no vegetarian or anybody else would think of using in a practical dietary.

Sometimes persons on changing from an ordinary flesh dietary, lose weight and strength. Generally, it is found that they have done little more than discontinue the flesh, without substituting suitable foods. Authorities think it is from a deficiency of proteid, and recommend an addition of such foods as pulse, wheatmeal, oatmeal, eggs, milk, cheese, and such as a reference to the table of analyses, show a low nutrient ratio figure. This may also be due to an insufficiency of food eaten, owing to the comparatively insipid character of the food and want of appetite. In making a change to a vegetarian diet, such foods had better be taken that are rather rich in proteid, and that approximate somewhat in their flavour and manner of cooking to that used previously. A further change to a simpler diet can afterwards gradually be made, according to conviction, tastes and bodily adaptability. It must not be expected that a change, even an ultimately very advantageous one, will always meet with an immediate and proper response from digestive and assimilative organs which have been accustomed for many years, perhaps by inheritance for generations, to another manner of living. There are several preparations produced from centrifugalised milk—that is milk from which the butter fat has been removed, which consist chiefly of proteid. These have a value in increasing the proteid contents of foods which may be thought deficient. The addition of these manufactured products appear unnecessary, as most of our food contains an abundance of proteid, and we can easily limit the quantity or avoid altogether those that are thought defective.

The later apologists for a flesh diet have had to admit that it is not a physiological necessity; but they have attempted to justify its use by a theory somewhat as follows. It is admitted, that any excess of proteid over that necessary for its special province of producing tissue, is utilised as a force-producer, in a similar manner to the carbo-hydrates. When the molecule is split up, and the carbon utilised, the nitrogen passes off in the form of urea by the kidneys. The theory propounded is that at the moment the nitrogen portion is liberated, it in some manner stimulates the living protoplasm of the nerve cells in its immediate neighbourhood to a higher state of activity. These views are given by Dr. Hutchison in his book on "Food," but there are no substantial grounds for them. It is only prompted by a wish to excuse a cherished habit. Sir William Roberts, M.D., in "Dietetics and Dyspepsia," p. 16 says that "high feeding consists mainly in a liberal allowance of meat, and in the systematic use of alcoholic beverages, and that low-feeding consists in a diet which is mainly vegetarian and non-alcoholic," and he proceeds to say that the high-fed classes and races display, on the whole, a richer vitality and a greater brain-power than their low-fed brethren. That "it is remarkable how often we hear of eminent men being troubled with gout, and gout is usually produced either by personal or ancestral high-feeding." We can only spare room for a few remarks on this subject. Intellectual and business ability brings wealth, wealth frequently leads to the pleasures of the table, but such habits are detrimental to sustained effort and clearness of mind. The children and grandchildren of such high livers are usually common-place, intellectually, and of deteriorated physique. The aristocracy who are generally high livers, notwithstanding their great advantages of education, travel and leisure, are not as a rule famed for their intellectual gifts. In the recent war the frugal living Japanese soldier has proved himself the most enduring and bravest in history; whilst the Japanese officers are more resourceful and tactful than the wealthier, high-fed Russian officers, with their aristocratic lineage. What is called high-feeding, is of the greatest benefit to the doctors and the proprietors of remedies for digestive and nervous disorders.

Food Adjuncts and Drugs.—In addition to the nutrients and the small quantity of indigestible fibre of which we have already written, food generally contains small quantities of substances which are difficult to classify, and whose action on the body is but imperfectly understood. Many of these possess pungent or strong odours and flavours. To them, various fruits, meats, etc., owe much of their characteristic differences of taste. When pure the proteids and starches are devoid of taste. Such oils and fats as are generally eaten have also but little flavour, providing they are free from rancidity and of good quality. The sugars differ from the other nutrients in possessing a more or less decided taste. The free vegetable acids also strongly affect the sense of taste, but they are only consumed in small quantities.

A drug may be defined as a substance which modifies the functions of the body or of some organ without sensibly imparting nourishment. This action may be one of stimulation or of depression. A drug is taken for its medicinal action, a food adjunct for its modifying action on food. It is impossible to give a quite satisfactory definition, or to draw sharp distinctions. For example, tea, coffee, alcohol and tobacco are sometimes placed in one group, and sometimes in another, according to opinion of their action and the definition of the terms food adjuncts, drugs and poisons. The difference of grouping often depends upon intensity rather than of kind of action. If taken frequently and not in quantity sufficient to have a markedly medicinal action, such things are generally called food adjuncts or supplementary foods, although much may be said in favour of a different view. The volatile oils of mustard, caraway, cloves, etc., are used in medicine; also the alkaloids of coffee and cocoa. Even honey is used as a mild laxative for infants; that is, as a drug. The difference between a drug and a poison is one only of degree. Some of the most esteemed drugs have to be administered in very small quantities, or they cause death; e.g., strychnine and morphine.

Classifications are necessary for methodical study, and for assisting the memory in grasping large numbers of things which can be grouped together. Classifications, however, are artificial, not due to natural lines of demarkation, but according to man's knowledge and convenience; hence a group is apt to approach and finally merge into another group, although on first consideration they appeared quite distinct. The disregard of this often leads to confusion and useless discussions.

Plants, like animals, as the result of tissue change, have certain used-up or waste matters to get out of the way. Animals have special excretory organs for the purpose; waste matter remains in the flesh and blood of dead animals. In plants are found a large number of powerful volatile oils, alkaloids, bitter resins, etc. Many of these are, in all probability, excretory products of no assimilative value to the plant. Certain volatile oils may attract insects, and in obtaining nectar from flowers insects assist fertilisation. Agreeable volatile oils and flavouring substances in fruits attract birds and animals. The eating of the fruits cause the seeds, which are uninjured by passing through the digestive system, to be disseminated over wide areas to the advantage of the plant species. On the other hand, nauseous and poisonous alkaloids, oils, resins, etc., serve as a protection against the attacks of browsing animals, birds, caterpillars, snails, etc. These nauseous substances are most abundant in the bark, husk, skin and outer parts. It is commonly supposed that the food on which each animal, including man, subsists, is especially produced by Nature for the purpose. This is an error, for each species of plant and animal lives for itself alone, and protects itself, with more or less success, against destruction by its competitors and enemies. Each species of animal selects from its surroundings such food as is most suitable. Such food may not be theoretically perfect; that is, it may not contain the maximum of nourishment free from innutritious matter; but during the long period of evolution, each species of animal has become possessed of organs suited to its environment. If to such animals be given food containing less indigestible matter, or food which is more readily digested by laboratory tests made independently of the living animal, their digestive system will be thrown out of gear, become clogged up or refuse to work properly, just as the furnace of a steam boiler, made to burn coal, will act badly with wood or petroleum. Many scientific men have overlooked this fact, and have endeavoured to produce food substances for general consumption, in the most concentrated and soluble form, thinking such food would be more easily assimilated.

The Volatile and Essential Oils are contained in minute quantity in a very large number of animal and vegetable foods. They contribute in part to the flavour of fruits. They are the cause of the pungency and aroma of mustard, horse-radish, cloves, nutmegs, cinnamon, caraway seeds, mint, sage and other spices. Onions contain a notable quantity. When extracted the essential oils become powerful drugs. In moderate quantities they are stomachic and carminative, in larger quantities irritant and emetic. Condiments and spices not only add flavour to food, but stimulate the secretion of gastric juice and peristaltic movement.

The Alkaloids most used are those of tea, coffee, kola-nut, cocoa, coca, tobacco and opium. Although the two last are generally smoked, they must be classed amongst the food adjuncts. It is of little consequence whether their active principles enter the body by the mouth and saliva or the lungs; their action on the blood and nervous system is the same.

The Extractives, as they are called, comprise a number of bodies of varying nature. They especially exist in flesh and flesh extracts. Amongst these are the purins. They will be treated at greater length hereafter.

Alcohol is to some extent a true food, but its stimulant and other action quite overshadows any food value it may possess.

There are other bodies such as the resins and bitters. The active principle of Indian hemp is a resin.

There is a great difference of opinion as to the extent to which stimulants may advantageously be used. It is remarkable that amongst nearly all nations, either alcohol in some form or one of the stronger alkaloids is in common use. From this fact it is sometimes argued that stimulants must supply a physiological need. The same method of reasoning will apply with greater force to the use of condiments. Such conclusions appear to us to be scarcely warranted. If the extensive or even universal practice of a thing proves its necessity, then has there been justification, either now or in the past, for war, lying, avarice and other vices. It is strange that drugs differing so greatly in their immediate and obvious effects as, for example, alcohol and opium, or coffee and tobacco should be used. Should it he said that only some of the much used stimulants are useful, there is an end to the argument based on their universal use. There is no doubt that the use of stimulants in more than very small quantities is distinctly injurious, and it is difficult to see what physiological advantage there can be in their habitual use, to what is vaguely called a moderate extent. Sometimes they are taken for a supposed medical necessity, and where taste attracts, little evidence satisfies. Those in the habit of taking them, if honest, must confess that it is chiefly on account of the apparent enjoyment. The ill-nourished and the depressed in body and mind crave most for stimulants. A food creates energy in the body, including the nervous system, and this is the only legitimate form of stimulation. A mere stimulant does not create but draws on the reserve forces. What was latent energy—to become in the natural course gradually available—under stimulation is rapidly set free; there is consequently, subsequent depletion of energy. There may occasionally be times when a particular organ needs a temporary stimulus to increased action, notwithstanding it may suffer an after depression; but such cases are so rare that they may be left out of our present argument, and stimulants should only be used, like other powerful drugs, under medical advice. In the last 25 years the use of alcohol by the medical profession has steadily diminished, its poisonous properties having become more evident.

There is a general similarity in the effects of stimulants on the digestive and nervous systems. The most largely used stimulant is ethyl alcohol, and as its action is best known, it may be useful to name the principal effects. Alcohol in the form of wine and spirits, in small quantities, first stimulates the digestive organs. Large quantities inflame the stomach and stop digestion. (Beer, however, retards digestion, altogether out of proportion to the alcohol it contains.) Alcohol increases the action of the heart, increases the blood pressure, and causes the vessels of the whole body to dilate, especially those of the skin; hence there is a feeling of warmth. It the person previously felt cold he now feels warm. The result of the increased circulation through the various organs is that they work with greater vigour, hence the mental faculties are brightened for a time, and the muscular strength seems increased. The person usually feels the better for it, though this is not always the case; some have a headache or feel very sleepy. It has been repeatedly proved that these good results are but transitory. The heart, although at first stimulated, is more exhausted after the action of the alcohol has passed away than it was at first. This is true of all the organs of the body which were stimulated. In consequence of the dilatation of the blood vessels of the skin, an unusual quantity of heat is lost and the body is cooled. After taking alcohol persons are less able to stand cold. When overtaken by snowstorms or subjected to excessive or prolonged cold, it has often happened that those who resorted to spirit drinking have succumbed, whilst the others have survived. Insurance statistics have conclusively shown that teetotallers are longer livers than the so-called moderate drinkers. The terrible effects on both body and mind of the excessive drinking of alcohol, or the use of other strong stimulants or narcotics, are too obvious to need allusion to here; we are only concerned with what is vaguely called their moderate use.

The stimulation produced by tea and coffee is in some respects like that of alcohol. The heart is stimulated and the blood pressure rises. The kidneys are strongly affected in those unaccustomed to the drug, but this ceases after a week or more of use. Their chief effect is on the brain and nervous system.

Many have boasted that they can take of what they call the good things of life to their full, without any bad effect, and looking over a few years, or even many years, it seems a fact. Some of us have known of such men, who have been esteemed for their joviality and good nature, who have suddenly broken down at what should have been a hearty middle life. On the other hand there are men who were badly equipped for the battle of life, with indifferent constitutions, who never had the buoyancy and overflow of animal spirits, but who with care have long outlived all their formerly more robust but careless companions.

Simple versus Highly-flavoured Foods.—It is very difficult to decide to what extent condiments and flavourings should be used. These have stimulating properties, although differing from the more complex properties of alcohol and the alkaloids. The great differences in the dietetic practices of nations does not appear to be in conformity with any general rule. It varies with opportunity, climate and national temperament; though doubtless the national temperament is often due in part to the dietetic habits. Some races are content with the simplest foods, large numbers subsist chiefly on rice, others on the richer cereals, wheat, oatmeal, etc., and fruit. On the other hand there are races who enjoy stronger flavoured food, including such things as garlic, curry, pickles, pepper, strong cheese, meat extracts, rancid fats, dried and smoked fish, high game or still more decomposed flesh, offal and various disgusting things. The Greenlanders will eat with the keenest appetite, the half-frozen, half-putrid head and fins of the seal, after it has been preserved under the grass of summer. In Burmah and Sumatra a mess is made by pounding together prawns, shrimps, or any cheap fish; this is frequently allowed to become partially putrid. It is largely used as a condiment for mixing with their rice.

Numerous examples of this sort could be given. There is scarcely anything that it is possible to eat, but has been consumed with relish by some tribe or other. The strongest flavoured, and to our minds most disgusting foods are eaten by the least intelligent and most brutal races. It is hunger that compels the poor African bushman to eat anything he can get, and the Hottentot not only the flesh, but the entrails of cattle which die naturally, and this last he has come to think exquisite when boiled in beast-blood. All this shows a wonderful range of adaptability in the human body, but it would not be right to say that all such food is equally wholesome. The most advanced and civilised races, especially the more delicately organised of them are the most fastidious, whilst it is the most brutal, that take the most rank and strongly flavoured foods. Even amongst the civilised there are great differences. The assimilative and nervous systems can be trained to tolerate injurious influences to a remarkable degree. A striking example is seen in the nausea commonly produced by the first pipe of tobacco, and the way the body may in time be persuaded, not only to tolerate many times such a quantity without manifesting any unpleasant feelings, but to receive pleasure from the drug. Opium or laudanum may be taken in gradually increasing quantities, until such a dose is taken as would at first have produced death, yet now without causing any immediate or very apparent harm. Nearly all drugs loose much of their first effect on continued use. Not only is this so, but a sudden discontinuance of a drug may cause distress, as the body, when free from the artificial stimulation to which it has become habituated, falls into a sluggish or torpid condition. For the enjoyment of food two things are equally necessary, a healthy and keen appetite and suitable food; without the first no food, however good and skilfully prepared, will give satisfaction. The sense of taste resides in certain of the papilloe of the tongue, and to a much less degree in the palate. Tastes may be classified into sweet, bitter, acid and saline. Sweet tastes are best appreciated by the tip, acid by the side, and bitter by the back of the tongue. Hot or pungent substances produce sensations of general feeling, which obscure any strictly gustatory sensations which may be present at the same time. To affect the taste the food must enter into solution. Like the other senses, taste may be rendered more delicate by cultivation. Flavours are really odours, and the word smell would be more appropriate. For example, what we call the taste of an onion, the flavour of fruit, etc. (independent of the sweetness or sourness of the fruit) is due to the nose.

Much has been written on the necessity of making food tasty, so as to stimulate the appetite and digestion. It is urged that unless this is done food will not be eaten in sufficient quantity. Innumerable receipts (some very elaborate) have been published for this purpose. All this is supposed to increase the enjoyment of food. The Anglo-Saxon race—the race whose dietary is the most elaborate —is especially subject to digestive derangements, and without good digestion and the consequent healthy appetite, no food will give full gustatory pleasure. The most wholesome food, and that which can be eaten most frequently without weariness, is mildly flavoured and simply prepared. Plain bread is an example; whereas sweet bread, currant bread, etc., though agreeable in small quantity, or as an occasional delicacy, soon palls on the appetite. Rice is the poorest and mildest flavoured of the cereals, it is therefore often, perhaps generally, made more tasty by the addition of fish, curry, etc. The bulk of the Chinese live on rice, with the exception of only 3 or 4 ounces of fish per day, and they are a fine, big and strong race. The Japanese labourer lives on similar food. In India rice is the food most in use, though many other cereals are eaten there. Other races live chiefly on fruits. It appears that the digestive organs will perform their functions perfectly with the mildest flavoured food. There is nothing surprising in this. The strongest, most intelligent, and largest animals are those which feed on grass, herbs and fruits. Even the African lion is no match for the gorilla. The lion and tiger are capable of great strength, but they cannot put it forth for long periods as can the herbivora. Our most useful animal, the horse, can exert much more muscular energy, weight for weight, than any of the carnivora. The cost of feeding one of the herbivora is much less than that of one of the carnivora of the same weight. This is so whether we take the cost of purchasing the food; or the expenditure of time, labour and energy on the part of man or of natural forces in the production of the food. Herbs, roots, corn and fruit are produced much more abundantly and freely than the corresponding quantity of sheep, deer, etc., on which the carnivora feed.

The restlessness, craving for novelty, and love of excitement, so characteristic of the Anglo-Saxon, and to a less extent of some other European races, has its correspondence in the food of these races. Highly-seasoned and nitrogenous foods act as a stimulant and favour spasmodic, and for a time perhaps, great intellectual and physical exertion, with a succeeding period of exhaustion. Simpler food favours long, sustained, uniform muscular strength, clearness of intellect, and contentment. Let no one misunderstand us; we do not assert that all who live on simple food have either clear intellects or are contented, because there are other factors besides food, but that such qualities are more easily retained or obtained under that condition. It is well known that the overfed and badly fed are the most irritable and discontented Those living on a stimulating dietary consisting largely of flesh have their chief successes in feats of short duration. Simple and abstemious living individuals or races excel in laborious work requiring endurance over long periods, such as long walking, cycling, and other athletic feats and long military campaigns.

The digestive and assimilative organs need the food constituents of which we have written, in proper proportion and quantity, and in a fairly digestible condition. Within these very wide and comprehensive limits, the organs can be trained. Very much of the great difference in food is due to the non-essential flavouring and stimulating part, rather than to that part which is essential and nourishing. What is the best, interests but few; whilst what is at present the pleasantest, influences the many. The ego, the superphysical conscious and reasoning entity should rule its material body, its temporary vehicle. The body, being the servant of the ego, just as a horse, dog, or other of the lower animals recognises its master, becomes a docile subject. The body can be led into good habits nearly as easily as into bad ones; often more easily, as bad habits are sometimes painfully acquired. The body being once habituated to certain movements, conditions, foods or drinks, within reasonable limits, derives pleasure therefrom and resists change. It is only when the food, etc., transgresses certain elementary principles, that the result is more or less painful. We may on scientific principles condemn flesh-foods, stimulants and elaborately prepared foods; but after ruling all this out, there is still left a very great variety of foods and methods of preparing them: hereon each individual must form his own opinion. Of the foods thus left, the same kind is not equally suitable to everyone, nor even to the same person at different periods.

A delicately balanced, fine-grained, high-toned mind and body responds to every tender influence, and is painfully jarred by that which is coarse. To such, fruits and delicately flavoured and easily digested foods are doubtless best and conducive to purity and clearness of thought. A coarse-grained, badly poised, roughly working body and spirit, is non-responsive except to loud or coarse impulses; and such a one's appetite is gratified, not by simple but by coarsely seasoned foods.

A person who is accustomed to a stimulating dietary of flesh-foods, especially if well-seasoned, finds a simple diet unsatisfying. Should such persons dine off simple vegetarian food, there is a tendency to over-eating. The less stimulating food fails to rouse the digestive organs and to appease the appetite; although an ample supply of nourishment be consumed. This is the reason why so many imagine that it is necessary to eat a larger quantity of food if it be vegetable. Should a distressing fulness and flatulence result from their over-feeding, they lay the blame to the vegetarian dietary instead of to themselves. Most persons, on changing to a vegetarian dietary, commence by imitating flesh dishes in appearance and flavour and even in the names. There is the additional inducement that the food may be attractive and palatable to friends who lack sympathy with the aesthetic and humane principles of the diet. After a while many of them incline to simpler flavoured foods. They revert to the unperverted taste of childhood, for children love sweets, fruits, and mild-flavoured foods rather than savouries. One who loves savouries, as a rule, cares much less for fruits. By compounding and cooking, a very great variety of foods can be prepared, but the differences in taste are much less than is usually, supposed. The effect of seasoning instead of increasing the range, diminishes it, by dulling the finer perception of flavours. The predominating seasoning also obscures everything else. The mixture of foods produces a conglomeration of tastes in which any particular or distinct flavours are obscured, resulting in a general sameness. It is often stated that as an ordinary flesh-eater has the choice of a greater range of foods and flavours than a vegetarian, he can obtain more enjoyment, and that the latter is disagreeably restricted. Certainly he has the choice, but does he avail himself of it to any considerable extent? No one cares to take all the different kinds of food, whether of animal or vegetable that are possible. Of edible animals but a very few kinds are eaten. A person who particularly relishes and partakes largely of flesh-foods will reject as insipid and unsatisfying many mild-flavoured foods at one end of the scale. The vegetarian may abstain from foods at the opposite end of the scale, not always from humane reasons, but because they are unpleasant. Thus there may be little to choose between the mere range of flavours that give enjoyment to each class of persons. The sense of taste is in its character and range lower than the sense of sight and hearing. The cultivation of the taste for savouries seems to blunt the taste for fruits and the delicate foods. The grass and herbs on which the herbivora subsist, seems to our imagination of little flavour and monotonous; but they eat with every sign of enjoyment, deliberately munching their food as though to get its full flavour. In all probability they find a considerable range of flavours in the great varieties of grasses commonly found together in a pasture.

Our elaborate cooking customs entail a vast amount of labour. They necessitate the cost, trouble and dirt from having fires in great excess of that required for warmth: the extra time in preparing, mixing and attending to food which has to be cooked: and the large number of greasy and soiled utensils which have to be cleaned. Cooked savoury food is generally much nicer eaten hot, and this necessitates fires and attention just previous to the meal. We have already said that soft cooked food discourages mastication and leads to defective teeth. Our elaborate cookery is mainly due to our custom of eating so largely of flesh, whilst the eating of flesh would receive a great impetus on the discovery of the art of cooking. Flesh can only be eaten with relish and with safety when cooked. Such a large proportion of it is infected with parasites, or is otherwise diseased, that it would he dangerous to eat it raw, even were it palatable in such a state. In those countries where man eats flesh in a raw or semi-cooked form, parasitic diseases are common. There is not the least doubt that our habit of eating so much cooked food is responsible for much over-eating, hasty eating, dyspepsia and illness. In regard to the making of bread, porridge, and many other comparatively simple prepared foods, the advantages of cooking seem overwhelmingly great. With our present imperfect knowledge and conflicting opinions, it is impossible to arrive at any satisfactory conclusion, and the whole question requires careful and impartial investigation. Experiments have been made with animals, chiefly pigs, with cooked and uncooked clover, hay, corn, meal, etc. (U.S. Department of Agriculture). It was found that the food was more or less diminished in digestibility by cooking. At least 13 separate series of experiments with pigs in different part of the country have been reported. In 10 of these trials there has been a positive loss from cooking the food. The amount of food required to produce in the animal a pound gain in weight was larger when the food had been cooked than when it was given raw. In some cases, the increased quantity of food required after cooking was considerable.

Those who live on uncooked food contend that a smaller quantity of nourishment is required. As uncooked food requires more mastication and is eaten more slowly, there is a better flow of saliva and time is given for the digestive organs to be gradually brought into complete action, and finally for the appeasing of the appetite. In the case of the members of the fruitarian family, whose food was uncooked, and of whom we have previously written, the quantity of nutriment taken was much less than that thought necessary, even after making full allowance for their small stature and weight.

Meat Extracts.—Justus von Liebig, the great German chemist, was the first to attempt to make these on the commercial scale. He described a method in

1847, and this not proving satisfactory, another one in 1865. He stated that the only practicable plan on a manufacturing scale, was to treat the chopped flesh with eight to ten times its weight of water, which was to be raised to 180° F. In another passage he says it is to be boiled for half-an-hour. After straining from all the undissolved meat fibre, etc., and carefully cleansing from all fat, the decoction is to be evaporated to a soft extract; such a preparation is practically free from albumin, gelatin and fat; all the nutritive principles except the saline matter having been extracted. Liebig states that 34 pounds of meat are required to produce 1 pound of extract. In 1872, he wrote "neither tea nor extract of meat are nutritive in the ordinary sense," and he went on to speak of their medicinal properties. Druit, in 1861, in describing the effect of a liquid preparation of meat, states that it exerted a rapid and stimulating action on the brain, and he proposed it as an auxiliary and partial substitute for brandy, in all case of great exhaustion or weakness attended with cerebral depression or despondency. In like manner, a feast of animal food in savages, whose customary diet was almost exclusively vegetable, has been described by travellers as producing great excitement and stimulation similar to that of intoxicating spirits. Similar effects have been observed from a copious employment of Liebig's extract. Voit asserts, from the results of his experiments, that extract of meat is practically useless as a food, and other authorities are quite of the same opinion, although they may value it as a stimulant and drug. _The Extra Pharmacopæia_, 1901, states that "Liebig's Extract or Lemco consists of creatin, creatinin, globulin and urea, with organic potash and other salts. It has been much over-estimated as a food either for invalids or healthy persons; still it is often valuable as a flavouring to add to soups, beef-tea, etc., and it is a nerve food allied to tea." Meat extracts stimulate the action of the heart and the digestive processes, but as in the case of other stimulants there is a succeeding period of depression. The *British Medical Journal* says that the widespread belief in the universal suitability of concentrated beef-tea is frequently responsible for increasing the patient's discomfort, and is even capable in conditions of kidney inefficiency, of producing positive harm. Some of the meat bases, the leucomaines, have been found to possess marked poisonous effects on the body. The manfacturers of meat extracts continue to mislead the public by absurdly false statements of the value of their products. They assert that their extracts contain the nutritive matter of 30, 40 or 50 times their weight of fresh meat, or that one or two meat-lozenges are sufficient for a meal. One company, asserts by direct statement, or imply by pictorial advertisement, that the nutritive matter in an ox can be concentrated into the bulk of a bottle of extract; and another company that a tea-cup full is equivalent in food value to an ox. Professor Halliburton writes: "Instead of an ox in a tea-cup, the ox's urine in a tea-cup would be much nearer the fact, for the meat extract consists largely of products on the way to urea, which more nearly resemble in constitution the urine than they do the flesh of the ox." Professor Robert Bartholow has also stated that the chemical composition of beef-tea closely resembles urine, and is more an excrementitious substance than a food. Those whose business it is to make a pure meat-broth, for the purpose of preparing therefrom a nutrient for experimenting with bacteria, cannot fail to recognise its similarity both in odour and colour to urine. Little consideration is needful to show the untruthfulness and the absurdity of the statements made by manufacturers as to the food value of these extracts. Fresh lean beef contains about 25 per cent. of solid nutriment and 75 per cent. of water. If lean beef be desiccated, one pound will be reduced to four ounces of perfectly dry substance; this will consist of about 80 per cent. of proteid matter and nearly 20 per cent. of fat including a little saline matter and the extractives. This is as far as it is possible to concentrate the beef. If it were possible to remove, without interfering with the nutritious constituents, the membraneous matter, the creatin, creatinine and purin bodies, we should reduce it to a little less than four ounces. It is very remarkable that the most nutritious matter of the beef, the muscle substance or proteid and the fat, are rejected in making Liebig's extract, whilst the effete or waste products are retained. In Bovril and some other preparations, some meat fibre has been added with the object of imparting a definite food value. Hence in some advertisements, now withdrawn, it was alleged that the preparations were immensely superior in nutritive value to ordinary meat extracts. The Bovril Company extensively circulated the following:—"It is hard for ladies to realise that the beef tea they make at home from the choicest fresh beef contains absolutely no nourishment and is nothing more than a slight stimulant. It is so, however, and many a patient has been starved on beef tea, whether made from fresh beef or from the meat extracts that are sold to the public. From these Bovril differs so much that one ounce of its nutritious constituents contains more real and direct nourishment than fifty ounces of ordinary meat extract." If analyses of meat extracts are referred to, it will be seen that the principal part of Bovril is the meat bases and other things common to all such extracts, and which the Company in their circular so emphatically condemn. If the meat fibre, which is the principal, if not the sole difference, is the only nourishing constituent, it is difficult to see the advantage over ordinary beef, which can be procured at a very small proportionate cost. Concerning this added meat fibre, C.A. Mitchell, in "Flesh Foods," writes: "As this amounts to at most some 8 or 10 per cent., it is obvious that a large quantity of the substance would be required to obtain as much unaltered proteid as is contained in an egg. On the other hand, it has been pointed out that there is nothing to show that flesh powder suspended in meat extract is more digestible than ordinary flesh in the same fine state of division, whilst the amount of flesh bases, the principal stimulating agents, is correspondingly reduced." Concerning added albumin and meat fibre, A.H. Allen, in "Commercial Organic Analysis," vol. iv., writes: "The amount of these constituents present in such a quantity of meat extract as is usually, or could be, taken at a time, is too insignificant to give it any appreciable value as nutriment." Notwithstanding such statements by analysts and others, Bovril is advertised to contain "the entire nourishment of prime ox-beef." The great extent of the extract of meat trade is shown by a circular issued by the Lemco and Oxo Company. They give the number of their cattle killed since 1865 as 5,550,000; stock of cattle 160,000; employees in works, farms and branches, 3,200. This is only one out of many such companies. It is a sad thing that myriads of animals should be slaughtered with all the horrible and brutalising surroundings of the slaughter-house to such a purpose—the nutritious matter being nearly all wasted. Reliance on these extracts is responsible for much sickness and death. Instead of their preventing colds, influenza, and other complaints as is professed, they predispose to them by overloading the body with waste products, taxing the excretory organs and reducing the vitality. The following analyses of meat extracts are by Otto Hehner:—

	Water.	Fat.	Gela-tin.	Albu-min.	Meat Fibre.	Albu-moses.	Pep-tones.	Meat Bases.	Ash.
Liebig Co.'s Extractum Carnis...	15·26	0·34	5·18	—	2·12	2·01	8·06	39·32	23·51
Armour's Extract of Meat	15·97	0·21	3·31	—	—	1·75	5·13	41·12	29·36
Brand & Co.'s Extractum Carnis	17·85	0·38	4·56	—	1·81	4·19	10·16	38·90	18·80
Brand & Co.'s Meat Juice	55·48	0·10	0·69	1·00	—	1·06	2·50	12·50	11·06
Brand & Co.'s Essence of Beef...	89·68	0·06	5·12	—	—	0·19	0·57	3·43	1·00
Valentine's Meat Juice	55·53	0·10	0·75	0·25	—	2·00	2·87	12·48	12·01
Bovril Company's Fluid Beef ...	28·34	1·02	3·81	—	5·37	8·38	13·18	19·38	17·67
Bovril for Invalids	24·34	1·07	4·56	—	5·87	5·56	6·44	34·07	16·50

Some of the "Liebig's Extract of Meat" so called, contains yeast extract; some even, is almost entirely, if not altogether made from yeast. The latter can be manufactured at a very low cost from brewers' and distillers' waste products, and there is a strong incentive for unscrupulous dealers to substitute it secretly. Artificial meat extracts prepared from yeast have the appearance and taste of meat extracts, but some, at least, have a considerably sharper flavour. In one method of manufacture common salt is added, and this renders it unfit for use in more than very small quantities as a flavouring. J. Graff has made analyses of ten yeast extracts, and contrasted them with meat extracts (see *Analyst* 1904, page 194), and says, "It will be seen that the chemical composition of yeast extract does not greatly differ from that of meat extract." Yeast extracts contain purin bodies, and are probably equally as injurious as meat extracts. Such strong and rank flavours (the odour is suggestive to us of putrefaction) should be discouraged by those who would cultivate a refined taste in food.

Flesh Bases and Waste Products.—As the result of destructive metamorphosis or the wearing out of the body, there remain certain waste products which have to be expelled as soon as is possible. Their retention and accumulation would soon produce death. A part is expelled by the lungs as carbon-dioxide, or as it is generally though less correctly termed, carbonic acid. Upon the breaking down of the complex proteid and other nitrogenous matter, the nitrogen is left in comparatively simple combinations. These effete nitrogen compounds are commonly termed flesh bases or nitrogenous extractives. They exist in small quantity in flesh meat, but are concentrated and conserved in the making of beef-tea or beef-extract. The spleen, lymphatic and other glands, and especially the liver, break these down into still simpler compounds, so that the kidneys may readily separate them from the blood, that they may pass out of the body. By far the largest part of this waste nitrogen is expelled from the bodies of men and many other mammals in the form of urea.

Pure urea is an odourless transparent crystalline substance, of cooling saline taste like nitre. It is soluble in an equal volume of water, and is expelled from the body with great ease. In the herbivora the nitrogenous waste takes the form of another body called hippuric acid. The nearly solid light-coloured urinary excretion of birds and serpents consists of urates; this is uric acid in combination with alkalies. In man, in addition to the urea excreted, there is also a little hippuric and uric acid or compounds of these. Uric acid is a transparent colourless crystalline body almost insoluble in water but soluble as urates in the presence of alkalies. As deposited from urine it is of a dull red sand-like appearance, as it has a great affinity for any colouring matter that is present.

It is only possible to make a brief reference to the chief organic bases. The xanthine bases are closely related to uric acid. Some of these occur in small quantity in the urine and animal tissues, others, such as caffeine, occur in plants. Creatine is a constant constituent of muscle substance. In fowl's flesh there is said to be 0.32 per cent., in cod-fish 0.17 per cent., and in beef 0.07 per cent. Creatinine is produced from creatine with great facility; it exists in urine. Both creatine and creatinine are readily soluble in water. A series of bases, closely allied to creatinine have been isolated from the flesh of large animals by A. Gautier; they are known as Gautier's flesh bases. When administered to animals, these act more or less powerfully on the nerve centres, inducing sleep and in some cases causing vomiting and purging in a manner similar to the alkaloids of snake venom, but less powerfully than the ptomaines. These bases are formed during life as a result of normal vital processes and are termed leucomaines.

Another class of bases of an alkaloidal nature, are termed ptomaines; these differ from the leucomaines, being produced by putrefactive or bacterial agency from dead flesh. The poisoning which has occasionally resulted from the eating of sausages, pork-pies, tinned meats, etc., is due to their having contained ptomaines.

Such quantities of waste products as are produced in the healthy body are excreted with ease, but it is otherwise in certain diseases. Either specially noxious substances are produced, or the usual substances are in excessive quantity and not eliminated with sufficient rapidity; in consequence the body is poisoned. Those who eat largely of flesh, introduce into their system the excretory matter contained therein, which super-added to the excretory matter resulting from the vital processes of the body puts an unusual and unnatural strain upon the liver and kidneys. It has been observed, that the eating of the flesh of some trapped animals has produced severe symptoms of poisoning. The pain and horror of having a limb bleeding and mangled in a most cruel steel trap, the struggles which only add to the misery, slowly being done to death during hours or even days of torture, has produced in their bodies virulent poisons. Leucomaine poisons have also been produced by the violent and prolonged exertions of an animal, fleeing from its pursuers, until its strength was completely spent. Cases are also known, where a mother nursing her infant, has given way to violent anger or other emotion, and the child at the breast has been made violently ill. We must not expect the flesh of any hunted or terrified animals to be wholesome. Animals brought in cattle ships across the Atlantic, suffer acutely. After rough weather they will often arrive in a maimed condition, some being dead. To this is added the terror and cruelty to which they are subjected whilst driven by callous drovers, often through a crowded city, to the slaughter house to which they have an instinctive dread. It is only to be expected that the dead flesh from such animals, should contain an unusually large quantity of the more poisonous flesh bases.

Purin Bodies.—The term purin has been applied to all bodies containing the nucleus C_5N_4. It comprises the xanthine group and the uric acid group of bodies. The principal purins are hypoxanthin, xanthin, uric acid, guanin, adenin, caffeine and theobromine. Purins in the body may either result from the wear and tear of certain cell contents, when they are called endogenous purins; or they are introduced in the food, when they are distinguished as exogenous purins. These purins are waste products and are readily converted into uric acid. The production of some uric acid by tissue change is, of course, unavoidable; but that resulting from the purins in food is under control.

An excess of uric acid is commonly associated with gout and similar diseases. The morbid phenomena of gout are chiefly manifested in the joints and surrounding tissues. The articular cartilages become swollen, with ensuing great pain. There is an accumulation of mortar like matter about the joints. This is calcium urate (not sodium urate as is generally stated). These nodular concretions are called tophi or chalkstones.

Very many are the hypotheses which have been propounded on the cause of gout and the part played by uric acid; many have had to be discarded or greatly modified. Though much light has recently been thrown on the subject, there remains much that is obscure. The subject is one which is surrounded with great difficulties, and would not be suitable for discussion here, were it not for the following reason: Certain views on uric acid as the cause of gout and several other diseases, are at the present time being pushed to the extreme in some health journals and pamphlets. Unfortunately many of the writers have very little knowledge, either of chemistry or physiology, and treat the question as though it were a simple one that had been quite settled. Our purpose is to clear the ground to some extent, for a better understanding of its fundamentals, and to warn against dogmatism. Our remarks, however, must be brief. It is undeniable that great eaters of meat, especially if they also take liberally of alcoholic drinks, are prone to diseases of the liver and kidneys, about or soon after the time of middle life. Flesh meat contains relatively large quantities of purins. Purins are metabolised in the body to uric acid, about half of the uric acid produced in the body disappears as such, being disintegrated, whilst the other half remains to be excreted by the kidneys.

One view is that whilst the organs of the body can readily dispose of its endogenous uric acid, or that produced by its own tissue change, together with the small amount of uric acid derived from most foods, the organs are strained by the larger quantity introduced in flesh-food or any other food rich in purins: that there is an accumulation in the system of some of this uric acid. Vegetable foods tend to keep the blood alkaline, flesh possesses less of this property; alkalinity of the blood is thought to be favourable to the elimination of uric acid, whilst anything of an acid nature acts contrarily. Dr. Alexander Haig writes "I consider that every man who eats what is called ordinary diet with butcher's meat twice a day, and also drinks acid wine or beer, will, by the time he is 50, have accumulated 300 to 400 grains of uric acid in his tissues, and possibly much more; and about this time, owing to the large amount of uric acid in his body, he will probably be subject to attacks of some form of gout or chronic rheumatism." Dr. Haig ascribes to the presence of uric acid in the system, not only gout and rheumatism, but epilepsy, hysteria, mental and bodily depression, diseases of the liver, kidneys, brain, etc.

The opinion of the majority of eminent medical men, during recent years, is that uric acid is not a cause, but a symptom of gout, that uric acid is not an irritant to the tissues, and that it is readily excreted in the healthy subject. Some of the reasons for this latter and against the previously stated hypothesis, are as follows:—Birds very rarely suffer from gout—the nodular concretions, sometimes found about their joints and which have been ascribed to gout, are of tuberculous origin—yet their blood contains more uric acid than that of man, and the solid matter of their excretion is mainly urates. If uric acid caused gout we should expect the disease to be common in birds. It is a remarkable fact that the waste nitrogen should be excreted in the form of uric acid or urates from such widely differing classes of animals as birds and serpents. Birds have a higher body temperature than man, they are very rapid in their movements and consume a large amount of food proportionate to their weight. They live, as it were, at high pressure. Serpents, on the other hand, have a low body temperature, they are lethargic and can live a long while without food. There is no obvious reason why some animals excrete urea and others uric acid. As uric acid is a satisfactory and unirritating form in which waste nitrogen is expelled from the body of the active alert bird, as well as from the slow moving reptile, it is surprising if a very much smaller quantity acts as a poison in man. Many physicians are convinced that uric acid is absolutely unirritating. Uratic deposits may occur to an enormous extent in gouty persons without the occurrence of any pain or paroxysms. Urates have been injected in large amounts into the bodies of animals as well as administered in their food with no toxic result whatever, or more than purely local irritation. The most careful investigations upon the excretions of persons suffering from gouty complaints, have failed to show uric acid in the excretions in excess of that in normal individuals, except during the later stage of an acute attack. There is an excess of uric acid in the blood of gouty subjects; some eminent medical men say it is in the highest degree probable, that this excess is not due to over production or deficient destruction, but to defective excretion by the kidneys. The excess may arise from failure of the uric acid to enter into combination with a suitable substance in the blood, which assists its passage through the kidneys. Under the head of gout are classed a number of unrelated disturbances in the gastro-intestinal tract and nutritive organs, whose sole bond of union is that they are accompanied by an excess of urates, and in well developed cases by deposits in the tissues. This is why there are so many different causes, curative treatments, theories, contradictions and vagaries in gout. There are good reasons for believing that uric acid is not in the free state in the body. In the urine it is in combination with alkalies as urates, perhaps also with some organic body. It has been shown that the blood of the gouty is not saturated with uric acid, but can take up more, and that the alkalinity of the blood is not diminished. The excess over the normal is in many cases small; it is said to be absent in some persons, and rarely, if ever reaches the quantity found in leukaemia. Leukaemia is a disease marked by an excessive and permanent increase in the white blood corpuscles and consequent progressive anæmia. Neither does the uric acid of gout reach the quantity produced in persons whilst being fed with thymus gland (sweetbread), for medical purposes. In neither of these cases are any of the symptoms of gout present. In the urine of children, it is not unusual to find a copious precipitate of urates, yet without any observed effect on them.

The symptoms of gout point to the presence of a toxin in the blood, and it is this which produces the lesions; the deposition of urates in the joints being secondary. This poison is probably of bacterial origin, derived from decomposing fæcal matter in the large intestine. This is due to faulty digestion and insufficient or defective intestinal secretions and constipation. This explains why excessive feeding, especially of proteid food, is so bad. The imperfectly digested residue of such food, when left to stagnate and become a mass of bacteria and putrefaction, gives off poisons which are absorbed in part, into the system. This bacterial poison produces headache, migraine, gouty or other symptoms. Because of the general failure of gouty persons to absorb the proper amount of nutriment from their food, they require to eat a larger quantity; this gives a further increase of fæcal decomposition and thus aggravates matters. The voluminous bowel or colon of man is a legacy from remote pre-human ancestors, whose food consisted of bulky, fibrous and slowly digested vegetable matters. It was more useful then, than now that most of our food is highly cooked. About a third part of the fæcal matter consists of bacteria of numerous species, though chiefly of the species known as the *bacillus coli communis*, one of the less harmful kind which is a constant inhabitant of the intestinal tract in man and animals. This species is even thought to be useful in breaking down the cellulose, which forms a part of the food of the herbivora. Flesh meat leaves a residue in which the bacteria of putrefaction find a congenial home. Poisons such as ptomaines, fatty acids and even true toxins are produced. It is believed that there exists in the colons of gouty persons, either conditions more favourable to the growth of the bacteria of putrefaction, or that they are less able to resist the effect of the poisons produced. It has generally been found that milk is a very good food for gouty patients. This seems due to its being little liable to putrefaction, the bacterial fermentation to which it is liable producing lactic acid—the souring of milk. The growth of most bacteria, particularly the putrefactive kinds are hindered or entirely stopped by acids slightly alkaline media are most favourable. This explains how it is that milk will often stop diarrhoea.

Dr. Haig condemns pulse and some other vegetable foods, because, he says, they contain uric acid. Pulse, he states, contains twice as much as most butcher's meat. Vegetable foods, however, contain no uric acid and meat but a very small quantity. The proper term to use is purins or nucleins. Dr. Haig has used a method of analysis which is quite incapable of giving correct results. Many vegetarians have accepted these figures and his deductions therefrom, and have given up the use of valuable foods in consequence. We therefore give some of the analyses of Dr. I. Walker Hall, from "The Purin Bodies in Food Stuffs." The determination of the purins has proved a very difficult process. Dr. Hall has devoted much time to investigating and improving the methods of others, and his figures may be accepted with confidence.

The first column of figures indicates purin bodies in parts per 1,000, the second column purin bodies in grains per pound:—

			Mutton	0.96	6.75
Sweet bread	0.06	0.4	Salmon	1.16	8.15
Liver	2.75	9.3	Cod	0.58	4.07
Beef steak	2.07	4.5	Lentils and	0.64	4.16
Beef Sirloin	1.30	9.1	haricots		
Ham	1.15	8.1	Oatmeal	0.53	3.45
Chicken	1.30	9.1	Peameal	0.39	2.54
Rabbit	0.97	6.3	Asparagus	0.21	1.50
Pork Loin	1.21	8.5	(cooked)		
Veal loin	1.16	8.14	Onions	0.09	0.06
			Potatoes	0.02	0.1

The following showed no traces of purins: white bread, rice, cabbage, lettuce, cauliflower and eggs. Milk showed a very small quantity, and cheese consequently must contain still less.

The researches of Dr. Hall show that the purins of food are metabolised or broken down by gouty patients, almost as well as by normal individuals, any slight retention being due to increased capillary pressure. A portion of the purins remain undigested, the quantity depending upon the particular purin and the vigour of the digestive organs. Two rabbits had the purin hypoxanthin given to them daily, in quantities which if given to a man in proportion to his weight, would have been 17 and 3 grains respectively. These rabbits showed malnutrition, and after death degenerative changes were visible in their liver and kidneys. Dr. Hall has made a large number of personal experiments, and says that when he has taken large doses of purin bodies—such as 7 grains of hypoxanthin, 15 to 77 grains of guanin or 7 to 15 grains of uric acid, apparently associated symptoms of general malaise and irritability have frequently appeared. In gouty subjects such moderate or small quantities of purins which are without effect on the healthy subject, may prove a source of irritation to the already weakened liver and kidneys.

Professor Carl von Noorden says of gout, "with regard to treatment we are all agreed that food containing an excess of purin bodies should be avoided, and those words embody almost all there is to be said as to dietetics. Alcohol is very injurious in gout. Salicylic acid is a dangerous remedy. Alkalies in every form are utterly useless." Dr. J. Woods-Hutchinson says, "the one element which has been found to be of the most overwhelming importance and value in the treatment of gout and lith¾mia, water, would act most admirably upon a toxic condition from any source; first, by sweeping out both the alimentary canal primarily, and the liver, kidneys and skin secondarily; and secondly, by supplying to the body cells that abundant salt-water bath in which alone they can live and discharge their functions." Dr. Woods-Hutchinson proceeds to state, that the one active agent in all the much vaunted mineral waters is nothing more or less than the water. "Their alleged solvent effects are now known to be pure moonshine." The value consists in "plain water, plus suggestion—not to say humbug—aided, of course, by the pure air of the springs and the excellent hygienic rules."

It is a common experience amongst rheumatic patients, that they cannot take lentils, haricots and some other foods; sometimes, even eggs and milk are inadmissible. This is not for the alleged reason that they contain purins, or as some misname it, uric acid; but because the digestive organs are unequal to the task. It will be seen, that although Dr. Haig's hypothesis of uric acid as a cause of gout and some other diseases is disputed by many eminent physicians, his treatment by excluding flesh and other foods which contain purins, and also pulse, which is difficult of digestion by the weakly, is a wise one. It has proved of the greatest value in very many cases.

Digestion and nutrition is a complex process, and it may be faulty at various stages and in several ways; there may be either deficient or excessive secretions or inaction. Thus there are exceptions, where gouty symptoms, including an excessive quantity of urates in the urine, have only been relieved by the giving up of milk foods or starch foods (see *Lancet*, 1900, I., p. 1, and 1903, I., p. 1059).

Those particularly interested in the subject of the purins and gout are referred to the lecture on "The meaning of uric acid and the urates," by Dr. Woods-Hutchinson, in the *Lancet*, 1903, I., p. 288, and the discussion on "The Chemical Pathology of Gout" before the British Medical Association at Oxford (see *British Medical Journal*, 1904, II., p. 740).

Dr. George S. Keith, in "Fads of an Old Physician," has a chapter on rheumatic fever; he says that the disease is much more common than it was fifty years ago. He has never met with it in the young or old except when the diet had consisted largely of beef and mutton, and this although he has been on the outlook for at least forty years for a case of the disease in a child or youth who had not been fed on red meat. He speaks of it as being exceedingly common in Buenos Ayres and Rosario in the Argentine Republic, amongst the young; and that it leads to most of the heart disease there. The amount of meat, especially of beef, consumed by old and young is enormous. The main evils there, were anæmia in children and neuralgia both in old and young. Dr. Haig relates how he suffered from migraine all his life, until the time of his discontinuing butchers' meat. As meat contains a comparatively large quantity of purins and other bodies called extractives, it is probable that such quantities have an injurious effect, quite apart from the question of uric acid production. That an excessive meat diet lessens the vitality of the body and pre-disposes to disease is undoubted, but opinions differ as to how the injury is brought about.

On thorough Mastication.—We have written at some length on the quantity and constituents of food required per day and have criticised the usually accepted standards. We have since read a valuable contribution to the subject by Mr. Horace Fletcher in his book, "The A.B.-Z. of our own nutrition" (F.A. Stokes & Co., New York). Ten years previous to the writing of the book, when of the age of 4, he was fast becoming a physical wreck, although he was trained as an athlete in his youth and had lived an active and most agreeable life. He had contracted a degree of physical disorder that made him ineligible as an insurance risk. This unexpected disability and warning was so much a shock, that it led to his making a strong personal effort to save himself. He concluded that he took too much food and too much needless worry. His practice and advice is, be sure that you are really hungry and are not pampering false appetite. If true appetite that will relish plain bread alone is not present, wait for it, if you have to wait till noon. Then chew, masticate, munch, bite, taste everything you take in your mouth; until it is not only thoroughly liquefied and made neutral or alkaline by saliva, but until the reduced substance all settles back in the folds at the back of the mouth and excites the swallowing impulse into a strong inclination to swallow. Then swallow what has collected and has excited the impulse, and continue to chew at the remainder, liquid though it be, until the last morsel disappears in response to the swallowing impulse. In a very short time this will become an agreeable and profitable fixed habit. Mr. Fletcher has been under the observation of several eminent scientific men. Professor R.H. Chittenden, of Yale University, in his report refers to the experiments of Kumagawa, Sivén, and other physiologists; who have shown that men may live and thrive, for a time at least, on amounts of proteid per day equal to only one-half and one-quarter the amount called for in the Voit standard (see p. 32), even without unduly increasing the total calories of the food intake. Such investigations, however, have always called forth critical comment from writers reluctant to depart from the current standards, as extending over too short periods of time.

Dr. Chittenden writes that he has had in his laboratory, for several months past, a gentleman (H.F.) who for some five years, practised a certain degree of abstinence in the taking of food and attained important economy with, as he believes, great gain, in bodily and mental vigour and with marked improvement in his general health. The gentleman in question fully satisfies his appetite, but no longer desires the amount of food consumed by most individuals. For a period of thirteen days, in January, he was under observation in Professor Chittenden's laboratory. The daily amount of proteid metabolised was 41.25 grammes, the body-weight (165 pounds) remaining practically constant. Analysis of the excretions showed an output of an equivalent quantity of nitrogen. In February a more thorough series of observations was made. The diet was quite simple, and consisted merely of a prepared cereal food, milk and maple sugar. This diet was taken twice a day for seven days, and was selected by the subject as giving sufficient variety for his needs and quite in accord with his taste. No attempt was made to conform to any given standard of quantity, but the subject took each day such amounts of the above foods as his appetite craved. The daily average in grammes was, proteid 44.9

(1.58 ounces), fats 38.0, carbohydrates 253.0, calories 1,606. The total intake of nitrogen per day was 7.19, while the output was 6.90. It may be asked, says Professor Chittenden, was this diet at all adequate for the needs of the body— sufficient for a man weighing 165 pounds? In reply, it may be said that the appetite was satisfied and that the subject had full freedom to take more food if he so desired. The body-weight remained practically constant and the nitrogen of the intake and output were not far apart. An important point is, can a man on such food be fit for physical work? Mr. Fletcher was placed under the guidance of Dr. W.G. Anderson, the director of the gymnasium of Yale University. Dr. Anderson reports that on the four last days of the experiment, in February, 1903, Mr. Fletcher was given the same kind of exercises as are given to the 'Varsity crew. They are drastic and fatiguing and cannot be done by beginners without soreness and pain resulting. They are of a character to tax the heart and lungs as well as to try the muscles of the limbs and trunk. "My conclusion, given in condensed form, is this: Mr. Fletcher performs this work with greater ease and with fewer noticeable bad results than any man of his age and condition I have ever worked with." "To appreciate the full significance of this report, it must be remembered," writes Professor Chittenden, "that Mr. Fletcher had for several months past taken practically no exercise other than that involved in daily walks about town." Sir Michael Forster had Mr. Fletcher and others under observation in his Cambridge laboratories, and in his report he remarks on the waste products of the bowel being not only greatly reduced in amount, as might be expected; but that they are also markedly changed in character, becoming odourless and inoffensive, and assuming a condition which suggests that the intestine is in a healthier and more aseptic condition than is the case under ordinary circumstances. If we can obtain sufficient nourishment, as Mr. Fletcher does, on half the usual quantity of food, we diminish by half the expenditure of energy required for digestion. By thorough mastication the succeeding digestive processes are more easily and completely performed. What is also of great importance is that there is not the danger of the blocking up of the lower intestines with a mass of incompletely digested and decomposing residue, to poison the whole body. Even where there is daily defæcation, there is often still this slowly shifting mass; the end portion only, being expelled at a time, one or more days after its proper period. All this improved condition of the digestive tract, leaves more vitality for use in other directions, a greater capacity for work and clearness of brain.

Professor R.H. Chittenden, in "Physiological Economy in Nutrition," writes: —"Our results, obtained with a great variety of subjects, justify the conviction that the minimum proteid requirements of the healthy man, under ordinary conditions of life, are far below the generally accepted dietary standards, and far below the amounts called for by the acquired taste of the generality of mankind. Body weight, health, strength, mental and physical vigour and endurance can be maintained with at least one-half of the proteid food ordinarily consumed."

From these and other considerations, we see that it is not only unnecessary, but inadvisable to diet ourselves according to any of the old standards, such as that of Voit, or even to any other standard, until they have been very thoroughly revised. We shall probably find that as the body becomes accustomed to simpler food, a smaller quantity of the food is necessary. The proportion of proteids to other constituents in all the ordinary, not over manfactured vegetable foods, such as are generally eaten, may be taken as sufficient. Several cookery books have been compiled in conformity with certain proteid standards and also with some more or less fanciful requirements; these give the quantities and kinds of food which it is imagined should be eaten each day. Theoretically, this should be calculated to accord with the weight, temperament, age and sex of the eater and the work he or she has to perform. The dietaries that we have seen have their proteid ratio placed unnecessarily high. This high proteid ratio can be got by the use of the pulses, but except in small quantities they are not generally admissible, and in some of the dietaries they are ruled out. The difficulty is got over by the liberal use of eggs, cheese and milk. To admit a necessity for these animal products is to show a weakness and want of confidence in the sufficiency of vegetable foods. Some of these cookery books are of use in sickness, especially as replacing those of the beef-tea, chicken-broth, jelly and arrowroot order. They provide a half-way stage between flesh and vegetable food, such as is palatable to those who have not quite overcome a yearning for flesh and stimulating foods. The liberal use of animal products is less likely to excite the prejudice of the ordinary medical practitioner or nurse. Possibly, also, a higher quantity of proteid may be required on first giving up flesh foods.

The Use of Salt.—One of the most remarkable habits of these times is the extensive use of common salt or sodium chloride. It is in all ordinary shop bread, in large quantity in a special and much advertised cereal food, even in a largely sold wheat flour, and often in pastry. It is added to nearly all savoury vegetable food, and many persons, not content, add still more at the time of eating. No dinner table is considered complete without one or more salt-cellars. Some take even threequarters of an ounce, or an ounce per day. The question is not, of course, whether salt is necessary or not, but whether there is a sufficient quantity already existing in our foods. Some allege that there is an essential difference between added salt and that natural to raw foods. That the former is inorganic, non-assimilable and even poisonous; whilst the latter is organised or in organic combination and nutritive. The writer is far from being convinced that there is a difference in food value. Some herbivorous animals are attracted by salt, but not the carnivora. This has been explained by the fact that potassium salts are characteristic of plants, whilst sodium chloride is the principal saline constituents of blood and of flesh. In their food, the herbivora take three or four times as much potash salts as the carnivora. Of course, the sodium chloride in the flesh of the herbivora and frugivora is obtained from the vegetable matter forming their food, and very few of them have the opportunity of obtaining it from salt-licks and mineral sources. They must have the power of storing up the sodium chloride from plants in sufficient quantity, whilst the potash salts pass away. There is no justification for saying that they are worse off by being deprived of salt. If the ape tribe can thrive without added salt why should not man? Bunge considers that a restriction to vegetable food causes a great desire for salt. Opposed to this, is the fact that certain tribes of negroes who cannot obtain salt, add to their vegetable food wood ashes or a preparation of wood ashes; this is chiefly potash. One preparation used in British Central Africa was found to contain about 21 per cent. of potassium chloride to only 0.5 per cent. of sodium chloride. It has been said that vegetarians consume more salt than those who take flesh food. We doubt this; we know of many vegetarians who have a strong objection to added salt, and have abstained from it for years. Some find that it predisposes to colds, causes skin irritation and other symptoms. At many vegetarian restaurants the food is exceedingly salty; the writer on this account cannot partake of their savoury dishes, except with displeasure. Nearly all who patronise these restaurants are accustomed to flesh foods, and it is their taste which has to be catered for. Flesh, and particularly blood, which of course, is in flesh, contains a considerable quantity of sodium chloride; and most flesh eaters are also in the habit of using the salt cellar. These people are accustomed to a stimulating diet, and have not a proper appreciation of the mildly flavoured unseasoned vegetable foods. Only those who have, for a time, discontinued the use of added salt, and lost any craving for it, can know how pleasant vegetables can be; even those vegetables which before were thought to be nearly tasteless, unless seasoned, are found to have very distinct flavours. It is then perceived, that there is a much greater variety in such foods than was previously imagined. It is commonly urged that salt and other condiments are necessary to make food palatable and to stimulate the digestive functions. We, on the contrary, say that condiments are the cause of much over-eating; and that if food cannot be eaten without them, it is a sign of disorganisation of the digestive system, and it is better to abstain from food until the appearance of a natural and healthy appetite. An excess of salt creates thirst and means more work for the kidneys in separating it from the blood prior to its expulsion. Even should it be admitted, that certain vegetables contain too little sodium salts, a very little salt added to such food would be sufficient; there is no excuse for the general use of it, and in such a great variety of foods. It is thought that some cases of inflammation of the kidneys originate in excessive salt eating; certain it is that patients suffering from the disease very soon improve, on being placed on a dietary free from added salt and also poor in naturally contained sodium and potassium salts. It is also possible to cause the swelling of the legs (oedema), to which such invalids are subject, to disappear and reappear at will, by withdrawing and afterwards resuming salt-containing foods. The quantity of one-third of an ounce, added to the usual diet, has after a continuation of several days, produced oedema. In one patient, on a diet of nearly two pounds of potatoes, with flesh, but without added salt, the oedemia disappeared and the albumin in the urine diminished. As potatoes are particularly rich in potash salts, this case is significant, as showing contrary to expectations, that such quantity as they contained had not the irritating effect of added common salt. Salt and other chlorides have been shown by several observers, to be injurious, not only in diseases of the kidneys, but also of the liver and heart. In these diseases the excess of salt is retained in the tissues, it causes a flow of fluid into them, and so produces oedema and favours the increase of dropsy. The good effect of milk in such diseases has long been known; it is probably due to its relative poverty in sodium and potassium chlorides. Even in the case of three healthy men, by an abrupt change from a diet extremely rich in chlorides to one deficient, they were able to reduce the body-weight by as much as two kilos. (4 lbs. 6 oz.); this was by the loss of an excess of water from their connective tissues. Sodium chloride diminishes the solvent action of water on uric acid and the urates; but potassium salts, on the contrary, do not, they may even increase the action. Although nearly all the medical experience recorded has to do with diseased persons, such cases are instructive; it is only reasonable to suppose, that more than a very small quantity of salt in excess of that natural to the food, is a source of irritation in the body, even of the ordinarily healthy individual.

Summary.—Enjoyment of food is dependent upon appetite quite as much as upon the nature of the food. Better a simple repast with good appetite than sumptuous fare with bad digestion. There is indeed a causal relationship between simplicity and health. The savage likes the noise of the tom-tom or the clatter of wooden instruments: what a contrast this is to the trained ear of the musician. Uncivilised man has little enjoyment of scenery or of animal life, except as in respect to their power of providing him with food, clothing or other physical gratification. What an enormous advance has taken place. In the case of the painter, his eye and mind can appreciate a wide range and delicacy of colour. Man has improved on the crab-apple and the wild strawberry. From a wild grass he has produced the large-grained nutritious wheat. Vegetables of all kinds have been greatly improved by long continued cultivation. In tropical and sub-tropical climates, where wild fruits are more plentiful, high cultivation is of less importance than in temperate regions. In sparsely inhabited or wild, temperate and cold regions, in times past, when deer and other animals were plentiful, and edible fruits few, flesh could be obtained at less labour; or such intelligence and industry as is required for the cultivation of fruits, cereals, and other foods scarcely existed. Flesh almost requires to be cooked to be palatable, certainly this much improves its flavour. The eating of flesh tends to produce a distaste for mild vegetable foods, especially if uncooked. In process of time, not only flesh but vegetable foods, were more and more subjected to cooking and seasoning, or mixed with the flesh, blood or viscera of the animals killed. Next, food was manufactured to produce a still greater variety, to increase the flavour, or less frequently to produce an imagined greater digestibility or nutritiveness. Man has taken that which seemed most agreeable, rarely has he been intentionally guided by scientific principles, by that which is really best. Only of late years can it be said that there is such a thing as a science of dietetics; although cookery books innumerable have abounded. Of recent years many diseases have enormously increased, some even seem to be new. Digestive disturbances, dental caries, appendicitis, gout, rheumatism, diabetes, nervous complaints, heart disease, baldness and a host of other diseases are due, in a great measure, to abuse of food. One of the most learned and original of scientific men, Professor Elie Metchnikoff, in his remarkable book on "The Nature of Man," referring to the variety of food and its complexity of preparation says that it "militates against physiological old age and that the simpler food of the uncivilised races is better.... Most of the complicated dishes provided in the homes, hotels and restaurants of the rich, stimulate the organs of digestion and secretion in a harmful way. It would be true progress to abandon modern cuisine and to go back to the simpler dishes of our ancestors." A few have lived to a hundred years, and physiologists, including Metchnikoff, see no inherent reason why all men, apart from accident, should not do so. Most men are old at 70, some even at 60; if we could add 20 or 30 years to our lives, what an immense gain it would be. Instead of a man being in his prime, a useful member of the community, from about 25 to 60 or perhaps to 70; he would have the same physical and mental vigour to 80 or 90 or even longer. This later period would be the most valuable part of his life, as he would be using and adding to the accumulated experience and knowledge of the earlier period.

Some, perceiving the mischief wrought by luxurious habits, urge us to go back to nature, to eat natural food. This is ambiguous. To speak of animals as being in a state of nature, conveys the distinct idea of their living according to their own instinct and reason, uninterfered with, in any way, by man. The phrase, applied to man, is either meaningless, or has a meaning varying with the views of each speaker. If it has any definite meaning, it must surely be the giving way to the animal impulses and instincts; to cast off all the artifices of civilisation, to give up all that the arts and sciences have done for man, all that he has acquired with enormous labour, through countless failures and successes, during hundreds of thousands of years, and to fall back to the lowest savagery—even the savages known to us use art in fashioning their arms, clothing and shelter, to the time when man was a mere animal. Civilised man is not only an animal, but an intellectual and spiritual being, and it is as natural for him to clothe himself as for a cow to eat grass. Our intellect has been made to wait on our animal nature, whilst our spiritual has lagged far behind. Animal food and all else of a stimulating character, stimulates the lower nature of man, his selfish propensities; whilst mild food makes it easier to lead a pure life. In the treatment of habitual drunkards in retreats, it has been found that a permanent cure is rare upon the usual abundant flesh dietary. Only by the use of vegetable food, particularly farinaceous, can a permanent cure be assured. The editor of the Clarion, Mr. R. Blatchford, or "Nunquam," has lately adopted a vegetarian diet. He remarks with surprise, that although he has been a heavy smoker for more than 30 years, using not less than eight ounces of tobacco a week, often two ounces in a day, he has found his passion for tobacco nearly gone. He has had to get milder tobacco, and is now not smoking half-an-ounce a day. He says "it does not taste the same; I am not nearly so fond of it." He finds, with regard to wine, that he now cannot drink it, "it tastes like physic." He writes: "These things have come upon me as a revelation. I begin to see that the great cure for the evil of national intemperance is not teetotal propaganda, but vegetarianism."

We have given reasons of a scientific character, for abstaining from flesh as food, but higher than these are those relating to ethics. Everything relating to the slaughter-house is revolting to a refined and humane person. In the great slaughter-houses of Chicago; in those huge hideous box-shaped buildings, five or six storeys high, about ten millions of animals are killed every year. They are treated as if they were bales of merchandise and as destitute of feeling. Bullocks are struck on the head with a mallet and let fall into the basement of the building. They are whilst stunned or half-stunned, at once strung up by their hind legs to some machinery, which moves them along, their heads hanging downwards. Regardless of their agony, men run after them to cut their throats, followed by others with great pails to catch the blood. Much of the warm blood is spilt over the men or on the floors; but this is of no consequence, if but a small fraction of a minute is economised. In a short time, whether the animal has bled long enough or not, it reaches the lowest and darkest and worst ventilated portion of the gloomy building, where it is disembowelled. The walls and floors are caked with blood, the place is filthy, there is no proper lavatory accommodation, everything both to eyes and nose is detestable. Even if the windows were kept clean, light could not penetrate into the centre of the buildings. Consequently a large part of the work is done by artificial light. Tuberculosis is prevalent amongst the workpeople living under such unsanitary conditions. Serious crime is much more common amongst them than amongst any other class.

We English-speaking people, who pride ourselves on our civilisation and religion; who call ourselves the followers of the gentle Jesus, the Prince of Peace; yet hunt, shoot, trap and torture animals for food sport and science. Our main reason for eating flesh is that of personal gratification. We are loath to admit that the lower animals have any rights. Those Eastern peoples who are adherents to the teachings of the gentle Buddha hold life sacred. Mr. H. Fielding, who lived many years amongst the simple-minded Burmese, says that though there is now no law against the sale of beef, yet no respectable Burman will even now, kill cattle or sell beef. No life at all may be taken by him who keeps to Buddhistic teaching, and this is a commandment wonderfully well kept. "He believes that all that is beautiful in life is founded on compassion and kindness and sympathy—that nothing of great value can exist without them. Do you think that a Burmese boy would be allowed to birds'-nest or worry rats with a terrier, or go ferreting? Not so. These would be crimes. That this kindess and compassion for animals has very far-reaching results, no one can doubt. If you are kind to animals, you will be kind, too, to your fellow-men."

By participating in any form of cruelty or injustice, not only to our fellow-men, but also to the lower animals, we retard our progress towards the higher life, the subtler forces in man cannot find their full expression and we are less responsive to spiritual influences.

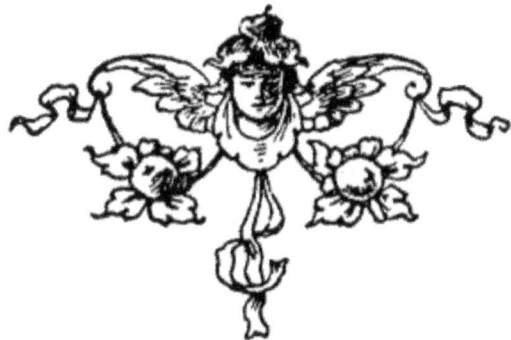

www.ingramcontent.com/pod-product-compliance
Lightning Source LLC
Chambersburg PA
CBHW080528030426
42337CB00023B/4662